HYDROXYCHLOROQUINE & IVERMECTIN -- MUCH MALIGNED SUPER DRUGS

HYDROXYCHLOROQUINE & IVERMECTIN -- MUCH MALIGNED SUPER DRUGS

BRIAN W. KELLY

Copyright © 2022 by Brian W. Kelly.

| ISBN: | Softcover | 978-1-6698-5150-9 |
| | eBook | 978-1-6698-5149-3 |

All rights reserved. No part of this book may be reproduced or transmitted in any form or by any means, electronic or mechanical, including photocopying, recording, or by any information storage and retrieval system, without permission in writing from the copyright owner.

Any people depicted in stock imagery provided by Getty Images are models, and such images are being used for illustrative purposes only.
Certain stock imagery © Getty Images.

Print information available on the last page.

Rev. date: 10/17/2022

To order additional copies of this book, contact:
Xlibris
844-714-8691
www.Xlibris.com
Orders@Xlibris.com
847562

LETS GO
PUBLISH!

CONTENTS

Dedication ix
Acknowledgments xi
Preface xiii
About the Author xv

Chapter 1   The Saga 1
Chapter 2   Origin 15
Chapter 3   The Virus Remedy Across the World! 22
Chapter 4   The World Declared a Lockdown! 31
Chapter 5   History of COVID-19—What Happened When? 37
Chapter 6   The "Cures" 69
Chapter 7   How to Resume Your Life 106
Chapter 8   Was the FDA's Hydroxy Decision based on Politics? 126
Chapter 9   Comments on the Goodness of Hydroxychloroquine ... 139
Chapter 10 Some HCQ Anecdotal Evidence 144
Chapter 11 That's Not All There Is 152
Chapter 12 The Hydroxychloroquine & Ivermectin Debate 162
Chapter 13 Is there a Scientific Consensus on Therapeutics? 167

Other Books by Brian W. Kelly 175

DEDICATION

I dedicate this book to all of the great health care workers and first responders. God bless you and thank you for your great assistance during the COVID-19 crisis

Thank You All!

ACKNOWLEDGMENTS

I appreciate all the help that I have received in putting this book together as well as all of my other 308 other published books.

My printed acknowledgments had become so large that book readers "complained" about going through too many pages to get to page one of the text.

And, so to permit me more flexibility, I put my acknowledgment list online, and it continues to grow. Believe it or not, it once cost about a dollar more to print each book.

Thank you and God bless you all for your help.

Please check out www.letsgopublish.com to read the latest version of my heartfelt acknowledgments updated for this book. FYI, Wily Ky Eyely loves this book and recommends it to all. Click the bottom of the Main menu on the web site!

Thank you all!

PREFACE

Why did Brian W. Kelly write this book?

Brian W. Kelly wrote this book because he cares about the United States and the other countries suffering from the pandemic today. I am publishing this book because I care.

I hope you enjoy this book and I hope that it inspires you to take the individual actions necessary to help yourself and all of us during this crisis. There are those in the limelight today that seem to be benefitting from imposing restrictions on American life. They do not seem to care whether their information is truthful or not. Government should be a helpful tool in solving this deep moral and potentially existential dilemma for our country.

So that you know, Brian Kelly is the most published non-fiction author in America with this, his 307th published book. Look it up, my dad is #1 and he writes over twenty books a year. Brian W., aka Brian Sr is not a health care specialist and has no medical training other than his own research. He is not a Doctor or in any way a mini-epidemiologist but he is well read like many who offer their worthwhile opinions on the many facets of the pandemic including the government's bias. Enjoy!

Ask everyone involved how they know the supposed truths which they pontificate. Prove them worthy of being recognized as being truthful or prove them as fraudulent. Your opinion counts in America. So does Brian Kelly's even though there are those who would like to shut him down and not let his words hit your ears.

I wish you the best.

Brian P. Kelly, Publisher
Wilkes-Barre, Pennsylvania

ABOUT THE AUTHOR

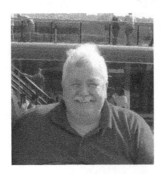

Brian W. Kelly retired as an Assistant Professor in the Business Information Technology (BIT) program at Marywood University, where he also served as the IBM i and Midrange Systems Technical Advisor to the IT Faculty. Kelly designed, developed, and taught many college and professional courses. He continues as a contributing technical editor to a number of IT industry magazines, including "The Four Hundred" and "Four Hundred Guru," published by IT Jungle.

Kelly is a former IBM Senior Systems Engineer and IBM Mid Atlantic Area Specialist. His specialty was designing applications for customers as well as implementing advanced IBM operating systems and software facilities on their machines.

He has an active information technology consultancy. He is the author of 309 books and numerous technical articles. Kelly has been a frequent speaker at COMMON, IBM conferences, and other technical conferences.

Brian was a candidate for US Congress from Pennsylvania in 2010 and ran for Mayor in his home town in 2015. He also ran in the primary for Congress in 2022. He brings a lot of experience to his writing endeavors. Losing several elections has taught Brian Sr. to approach life with humility.

Brian Kelly knows that the crisis can be solved with the right therapeutic in the short term. Keep the faith, we'll be on the streets soon.

CHAPTER 1

The Saga

Tell me about the problem?

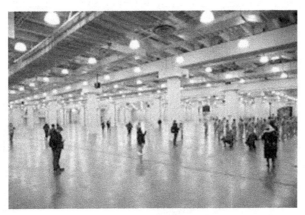

Javits Center, NYC Temporarily converted to a 2900 bed hospital

On March 11, 2020, After finding more than 118,000 cases in 114 countries and 4,291 deaths, the WHO declared COVID-19 a pandemic. Today we have had over 620 million cases worldwide and we are approaching 7 million deaths worldwide. In the US, we have had almost 100 million cases and over 1.1 million deaths. The Coronavirus was and still is a powerful force with which to be reckoned. Unfortunately it has become one of the biggest political footballs for political play. Try to find the truth about anything.

From the moment the focus of the world went to COVID-19, researchers across the globe have been searching for a cure and there are many supposed cures but which ones work? That is why many people across the globe feel they could use their own personal COVID expert to ferret through the information on the preventions and the cures. This book is one such source but the best bet is always to trust your local family doctor and take the action he or she recommends if you are infected. Also, it is good to ask advice on how you might be able to prevent getting the disease in the first place.

Researchers from the CDC found evidence that cases of COVOD-19 were found in December 2019, weeks earlier than previously thought—even before the first cases in Wuhan China had been publicly identified. From the time of first discovery, searches for cures were taking place wherever it was found.

Moving on the time line, in April 2020, the Washington Times wrote an article about an international poll of more than 6,000 doctors that found that the antimalarial drug hydroxychloroquine at the time was the most highly rated treatment for the novel coronavirus. Ivermectin was found to be effective in studies in 2021.

Coronavirus disease 2019 (COVID-19) is defined as an illness caused by a novel coronavirus now called severe acute respiratory syndrome coronavirus 2 (SARS-CoV-2; formerly called 2019-nCoV). The virus was first identified amid an outbreak of respiratory illness cases in Wuhan City, Hubei Province, China. In March 2020, the World Health Organization (WHO) declared the COVID-19 outbreak a pandemic. And the world has been fighting it to this day. Some believe that the fight takes place with many of the fighters having their hands tied behind their backs.

The survey that comprised the international poll of more than 6,000 doctors was conducted by Sermo, a global health care polling company, of 6,227 physicians in 30 countries found that 37% of those treating COVID-19 patients rated hydroxychloroquine as the "most effective therapy" from a list of 15 options. Despite this early opinion on the part of physicians worldwide.

Since April 2020, almost two and a half years have passed without a consensus or a definitive trial that all scientists and epidemiologists can sign off as correct. Some suggest that a negative verdict on Hydroxychloroquine is being promoted by many in the medical community and Big Pharma because this cure has been used effectively for other illnesses from 1940 and because it is easy to make, it may be too cheap for Bog Pharma to adopt.

The same goes for Ivermectin which came available in 197,5 though many physicians who actually treat COVID patients still swear by both of these two therapeutics. There is little room for big profits with these old time medicines. This is just opinion as there is no court of last resort to which to plead the case. But money often drives research.

Of the physicians surveyed, 3,308 said they had either ordered a COVID-19 test or had been involved in caring for a coronavirus patient, and 2,171 of those responded to the question asking which medications were most effective.

Sen. Ron Johnson, a Wisconsin Republican, sent then President Trump a letter when this survey was released. His letter was from more than 700 physicians urging him to expand the use of Hydroxychloroquine for coronavirus outpatients by removing federal and state restrictions limiting the drug's use to hospitals. Some may say that is not compelling evidence that Hydroxychloroquine has the efficacy to cure COVID-19 from infected persons but it sure is a major testimony from those who may know best. The fact that it is too cheap to adopt keeps ringing in my head.

Johnson said he forwarded the request to the White House after gaining support from 776 physicians, just 14 hours after he began circulating the letter, which asked Mr. Trump to issue presidential directives allowing doctors to "fight with all the weapons we have at hand."

The US Center for Disease Control has been working overtime for most of 2020 and 2021 and even part of 2019 and still into 2022, in response to the pandemic of a respiratory disease spreading from person-to-person. The source has been known for a long time. It is caused by a novel (new) coronavirus. There have been other coronaviruses but this one is different and it has received more attention than any virus in recent history. It is still on the big problem list for epidemiologists as it keeps changing its shape.

As previously noted, the disease has been named "coronavirus disease 2019" (abbreviated "COVID-19"). It comes with a very serious public health risk. The federal government of the US is very concerned for the safety of US citizens and has been working closely with state, local, tribal, and territorial partners, as well as public health partners, to respond to this bleak situation. COVID-19 can cause mild to severe illness; most severe illness occurs in adults 65 years and older. For some reason it creates a fatal situation in many adults over 65 years of age.

The United States still is the leader of cases in the world. This chart is representative but the numbers are higher as we wrap u 2022.

Number of novel coronavirus (COVID-19) deaths worldwide as of August 13, 2021, by country

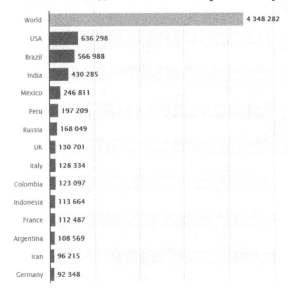

The worldwide death toll is approaching 700 million with over 100 Million cases. The US has over 100 million cases and 1.1 million deaths. It began slowly in the US and as soon as President Trump saw its lethality, and its origin in China, he cut off all travel to China and later Europe and then Great Britain. Why? It was his way of keeping the virus from our shores. Since that time, different parts of the US have been experiencing different levels of COVID-19 activity.

The United States nationally is affected by the yoyo nature of infections-up and down, down & up. The US was one of the first to come out of the acceleration phase of the pandemic. The duration and severity of each pandemic phase can vary depending on the characteristics of the virus and the public health response. In 2021, multiple strains of the virus have been more or less terrorizing many countries as the unknown contagion and strength of the new strains are a major cause of concern in most countries,

There have been times in which the model projections have the infection and death curves flattening meaning the virus had been substantially but not entirely mitigated.

CDC and state and local public health laboratories have been continually testing for the virus that causes COVID-19. Nonetheless it is still with us despite all the vaccinations and it looks like it will be with us for the long haul in various forms That does not mean that we should permit government to shut down the country again.

Consequently therapeutics such as remdesivir and hydroxychloroquine (2020), Ivermectin, (2021) and others (2022) are receiving more and more attention. The disease would not be as scary if there were a therapeutic accepted by all of science that could cure it post haste. More and more trials and truth in reporting results may be the best answer for America. Do not rule out Hydroxychloroquine as in my own family, it has been a godsend.

CDC Recommendation

With well over 98 million cases and over 1.1 million deaths as we close out 2022, in the US, and with the # of the cases increasing continually in recent weeks, the experts continue to blame newer highly transmissible coronavirus variants all the time. It is tough to keep up with the current score.

Modeling shows that the typical variant normally eclipses the other variants and accounts for more than 90 percent of new infections, according to data from the Centers for Disease Control and Prevention.

CDC Director Rochelle Walensky a while ago described the delta variant as a very different virus than the one that took hold in 2020. She said it was capable of generating infections even among vaccinated people, though those are likely to be far less severe. "The delta variant was showing every day its willingness to outsmart us and to be an opportunist in areas where we have not shown a fortified response against it," she said in July, 2021. More variants Thus the idea of a cure in the form of a therapeutic, even if it were hydroxychloroquine would be welcome indeed. Yet, the CDC does not work hard to prove or disapprove the two staples Hydroxychloroquine and Ivermectin despite much positive evidence.

After Delta came the Omicron strain (BA.1). It was first identified in Botswana and South Africa in late November 2021, and cases quickly began to surface and multiply in almost all countries including the US. other countries. At the end of August 2022, one of those subvariants, BA.5, made up more than 88% of cases in the United States, making it the predominant variant in this country. A related variant, BA.4, was also on the rise, making up about 8% of cases.

The original strain of Omicron was more transmissible than Delta was. One explanation was that more than 30 of Omicron's mutations are on the virus's spike protein, the part that attaches to human cells, and several of those are believed to increase the probability of infection.

Despite the fact that the major US agencies such as the NIH and the CDC and all of the apostles and prophets of epidemiology such as Dr. Anthony Fauci are implicitly trusted by the Biden Administration, with all the negative reporting Fauci and the CDC have both lost tons of credibility with the American people. When people with four vaccinations get the virus, fewer people trust those like Fauci who claim that vaccinations prevent catching the bug.

To answer the why question, consider all of the regular flip flopping advice they offer the people. So nobody in the body public trusts what to believe or not believe. The government is seen as having a stake in the issue and it is no longer trusted by many Americans.

The experts make recommendations and offer many precautions such as to mask or not to mask, indoors or outdoors. One day it is no masks, the next day it is any mask –even coffee filters, the days after it is two or three cloth masks. Children must be masked then not. Children are then not resistant to the disease.

Then everyone over two years of age needs vaccinations etc. etc. etc. Moreover, the public has caught on to the officials conducting a war on hydroxychloroquine because Trump liked it, rather than taking the time to really determine its efficacy. By now, after more than two and a half years of COVID, all therapeutics should have had their trials and the good and the bad should have been determined. Instead politics seems to guide the major agencies. The public suspects that all data freely given by government sources is worthless.

The CDC suggests that everyone can do their part to help the country respond to this emerging public health threat. Here are some of the CDC's important guidelines to which all Americans are asked to adhere.

The CDC recommendations and those of Dr. Fauci, who is supposedly retiring in a few months are for individuals to use a cloth face covering to keep people who are infected but do not have symptoms from spreading COVID-19 to others.

The cloth face cover is meant to protect other people in case you are infected and it offers some protection for you from others. The cloth face coverings recommended for the general population are not surgical masks or N-95 respirators. Other experts say only N-95 masks offer any protection but they are cost prohibitive. They argue that medical face masks such as N-95 are critical supplies that should be reserved for healthcare workers and other first responders, as recommended by CDC. If the supply of the N-95 were adequate in the US, there would be no restrictions on the type of face covering for individuals who are not part of a medical team.

Then we hear that the cloth face cover is not a substitute for social distancing, the primary means that the US is deploying to stop the spread of the virus. The CDC continues to recommend that people try keep about 6 feet between themselves and others even though the scientists use 3 feet as the proper distance. The story is never the same from two sources. What are the people to think?

You may recall that the White House's original "Slow the Spread" guidelines came after the 15-day shutdown and were to be in place temporarily. But the Democrats got power hungry with lockdowns and bossing the people around. These were part of the nation's effort to slow the spread of COVID-19 through the implementation of social distancing at all levels of society. Democrats decided lockdowns and shutting down restaurants was the answer but this merely put many in a vast # of job types out of work while doing little for the spread of the disease.

People 65 years and older and people with severe underlying medical conditions are still asked to take special precautions because they are at higher risk of developing serious COVID-19 illness. The death rate is substantially higher for elderly patients. Now with the delta and other variants, it is no longer good enough just to be vaccinated. No wonder why the people are confused.

If you are a healthcare provider, you are asked to use your judgment to determine if a patient has signs and symptoms compatible with COVID-19 and whether the patient should be tested. There are now plenty of tests so there is no reason for anyone suspecting COVID, to not be tested to make sure one way or another. Originally tests were in short supply but this situation has been solved. The sooner COVID is diagnosed, the better the chance of a quick recovery.

Those people who get a fever or cough should consider whether they might have COVID-19, depending on where they live, their travel history or other exposures. All of the U.S. has been seeing some level of community spread of COVID-19. Testing for COVID-19 may be accessed through medical providers or public health departments, but the experts still say there is no treatment for this virus.

Both Hydroxychloroquine and Ivermectin have always shown major promise as a prophylaxis (preventative) and as a cure for the virus. However because the topic is fraught with politics, it is my opinion that people are suffering and dying needlessly because the experts are concerned more about politics than about what's best for the people

Regular Use of Ivermectin as Prophylaxis for COVID-19 led up to a 92% Reduction in COVID-19 Mortality Rate in a Dose-Response Manner. These results came from a prospective observational study of a strictly controlled population of 88,012 subject. The study was recently published in August 31, 2022. Still no major US agency endorses it.

Because of the political nature of the controversy on the drug, there are no officially confirmed studies of the effectiveness of Hydroxychloroquine or Ivermectin. Yet, in hospital study after hospital study, early treatment helps big time. The first thing I would want I know, if I were infected with the disease would be Hydroxychloroquine with zincand vitamins and some Ivermectin with Vitamin D, Vitamin A, and in some cases, Azithromycin. My opinion of the most important element of that cocktail is the Hydroxychloroquine and Ivermectin. I have seen it work. But please ask your doctor first.

By the way, Azithromycin is a licensed, widely available, cheap, and generally safe drug that has been proposed as a treatment for COVID-19, with in-vitro studies suggesting activity against some viruses, including SARS-CoV-2. In other words, it helps and is worth taking as part of a cure cocktail as recommended by a physician.

Despite the limitations of doctor's prescribing hydroxychloroquine et al, doctors more concerned about making patient's well than appealing to the politics of the matter, treat patients with the best remedy possible and to many physicians—not covered by the general press, that remedy is none other than hydroxychloroquine. Recently the same positive press has been associated with Ivermectin.

Consequently, in many areas of the country, great and caring doctors use these drug to mitigate the COVID-19 disease and bring along a better outcome for their patients. And, why not?

The good news is that most people have mild illness with the disease and are able to recover at home without medical care. Some have major illnesses however, and do need hospitalization. Many experts believe that almost everybody has some level of herd immunity and the cases are less severe all the time leading people to grin and bear it like it is a cold. There is no better immunity that natural immunity from having had the virus.

If you are returning from a country with travel restrictions, you should stay home and monitor your health. All other international travelers please follow CDC instructions during this time. Your cooperation is integral to the ongoing public health response to try to slow spread of this virus.

The complete clinical picture with regard to COVID-19 is not fully known. The same can be said of the use of Hydroxychloroquine or Ivermectin as a therapeutic to address the reported illnesses. COVID-19 of course come sometimes as a very mild illness, including some cases in which there are no reported symptoms, to severe, including illness resulting in death. It is nothing to take lightly. While information so far suggests that majority of COVID-19 illnesses are mild. About 16% of the cases reported from China from the beginning were very serious.

A CDC Morbidity & Mortality Weekly Report that looked at severity of disease among COVID-19 patients in the United States by age group found that 80% of early deaths were among adults 65 years and older with the highest percentage of severe outcomes occurring in people 85 years and older. People with serious underlying medical conditions — like serious heart conditions, chronic lung disease, obesity, and diabetes, for example — also seem to be at higher risk of developing serious COVID-19 illness.

The COVID-19 is still an official pandemic though President Biden has euphemistically called it off—but not officially. FYI, a pandemic is a global outbreak of a disease. Pandemics happen when a new virus emerges to infect people and can spread between people sustainably. Because there is little to no pre-existing immunity against the new virus, it spreads worldwide. We have seen how devastating the results are. On top of that, the response of government officials with demands for behavior changes among the population, are deemed by many as more damaging to the country than the disease itself.

The virus that causes COVID-19 has been infecting people for well over a year with intermittent breaks. It has been spreading very easily from person-to-person. On March 11, 2020, the COVID-19 outbreak was labeled a pandemic by the World Health Organization (WHO). After what we have seen in the US< few take issue today with that label for the disease. It has been devastating for all countries.

This is the first pandemic known to be caused by this new coronavirus. In the past century, there have been four pandemics caused by the emergence of new influenza viruses. As a result, most research and guidance around pandemics is specific to influenza, but the same premises can be applied to the current COVID-19 pandemic.

Pandemics of respiratory disease follow a certain progression outlined by the CDC. They begin with an investigation phase, followed by recognition, initiation, and acceleration phases. The peak of illnesses occurs at the end of the acceleration phase, which is followed by a deceleration phase, during which there is a decrease in illnesses.

Different countries or parts of countries can be in different phases of the pandemic at any point in time and different parts of the same country can also be in different phases of a pandemic.

Risk Assessment

Risk depends on characteristics of the virus, including how well it spreads among people; the severity of resulting illness; and the medical or other measures available to control the impact of the virus (for example, vaccines or medications that can treat the illness). There are no vaccines or medications specifically intended to fight this virus.

In the absence of vaccine or treatment medications, non-pharma-ceutical interventions become the most important response strategy. These are community interventions that can reduce the impact of disease.

The risk from COVID-19 to Americans can be broken down into risk of exposure versus risk of serious illness and death.

Risk of exposure:

Cases of COVID-19 and instances of community spread are being reported in all states for the duration of the pandemic.

People in places where ongoing community spread of the virus that causes COVID-19 has been reported are at elevated risk of exposure, with the level of risk dependent on the location.

Healthcare workers actively caring for patients with COVID-19 have been proven to be at an elevated risk of exposure. Close contacts of persons with COVID-19 also are at elevated risk of exposure.

Travelers returning from affected international locations where community spread is occurring also are at elevated risk of exposure, with level of risk dependent on where they traveled.

Risk of Severe Illness:

Based on currently available information and clinical expertise, older adults and people of any age who have serious underlying medical conditions might be at higher risk for severe illness from COVID-19. Based on what we know now, those at higher risk for severe illness from COVID-19 are:

- People 65 years and older
- People who live in a nursing home or long-term care facility
- People of all ages with underlying medical conditions

Regardless of all of the above, there is no denying that besides an effective vaccine, the best solution would be to have a cure for the disease once contracted. Then it would not be so scary. There is a puzzlement among the people, however, who have been witnessing the politicization of various potential cures because they are favored by people from a different political way of thinking. That is to bad for the country that when the health of Americans lie in the balance, officials get their guidance from political expediency. America can do better than that for sure.

CHAPTER 2

Origin

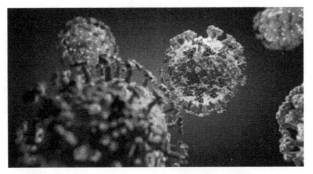

Coronavirus illustration (stock image).
Credit: © pinkeyes / Adobe Stock

On March 17, 2020, Scripps Research released a press release explaining the origins of the COvid-19 pandemic that the world has been enduring since even prior to the report, Much of the information in this chapter has been culled from their report as well as that from genengnews.com

On March 19, Geneng News put out a report that discussed the origins of the Coronavirus. In it they posture that the virus evolved naturally, and 'Is Not a Laboratory Construct.' This was proven by their genetic study.

Who do we trust?

What is the official name and why?

Official names have been announced for the virus responsible that is responsible for COVID-19. (It had previously been known as "2019 novel coronavirus") and the disease it causes. The official names are shown on the next page:

> **Disease name**
> coronavirus disease name is (COVID-19)

Virus name
Severe acute respiratory syndrome coronavirus 2 is (SARS-CoV-2)

The term *Novel* is used with this and means the following in this book:

Novel: *new and not resembling something formerly known or used.*

Why do the virus and the disease have different names?

Viruses, and the diseases they cause, often have different names. For example, HIV is the virus that causes AIDS. People often know the name of a disease, but not the name of the virus that causes it.

There are different processes, and purposes, for naming viruses and diseases.

Viruses are named based on their genetic structure to facilitate the development of diagnostic tests, vaccines and medicines. Virologists and the wider scientific community do this work, so viruses are named by the <u>International Committee on Taxonomy of Viruses (ICTV)</u>.

Diseases are named to enable discussion on disease prevention, spread, transmissibility, severity and treatment. Human disease preparedness and response at a world level right now is the role of the World Health Organization (WHO), so diseases are officially named by WHO in the International Classification of Diseases (ICD).

Origin of the disease and virus

The novel SARS-CoV-2 coronavirus emerged from the city of Wuhan, China, in late 2019. It has since caused a large scale COVID-19 epidemic (declared a pandemic on March 11, 2020) and it has spread to all of the 195 countries and territories as of October 6, 2022. This disease is the product of natural evolution, according to findings published recently in the journal Nature Medicine. Though this is current mainstream theory, some doubt its accuracy and believe it was a lab accident in Wuhan.

The analysis of public genome sequence data from SARS-CoV-2 and related viruses found no evidence that the virus was made in a laboratory or otherwise engineered. Despite this analysis, pundits across the world have voiced suspicion with the proximity of the outbreak to a large lab in the Wuhan province.

Though early indications were that the source was the Wuhan Wet markets, further information has become available that the virus may have escaped from one of the two labs in Wuhan. Though the source of the virus is likely the labs, there is no evidence to suggest that the virus is man-made. The official word is that the disease and the virus are the product of nature and were not manufactured for bio-war purposes. Here's how the scientists know.

"By comparing the available genome sequence data for known coronavirus strains, we can firmly determine that SARS-CoV-2 originated through natural processes," said Kristian Andersen, PhD, an associate professor of immunology and microbiology at Scripps Research and corresponding author on the paper.

In addition to Andersen, authors on the paper, "The proximal origin of SARS-CoV-2," include Robert F. Garry, of Tulane University; Edward Holmes, of the University of Sydney; Andrew Rambaut, of University of Edinburgh; W. Ian Lipkin, of Columbia University.

What are Coronaviruses?

Coronaviruses are a large family of viruses that can cause illnesses ranging widely in severity. The first known severe illness caused by a coronavirus emerged with the 2003 Severe Acute Respiratory Syndrome (SARS) epidemic in China. A second outbreak of severe illness began in 2012 in Saudi Arabia with the Middle East Respiratory Syndrome (MERS).

On December 31 of last year, Chinese authorities alerted the World Health Organization of an outbreak of a novel strain of coronavirus causing severe illness. This was subsequently named SARS-CoV-2. As of Oct 6, 2022, the US and Pennsylvania Stats are as follows:

United States Stats
Cases: 100 million
Deaths: 1.1 million

Pennsylvania Stats
Cases: 3.3 million
Deaths: 48,000

What do we know now about the disease and the virus?

Very shortly after the epidemic began, Chinese scientists sequenced the genome of SARS-CoV-2 and made the data available to researchers across worldwide. Let me explain how significant this was.

Two biologists from John Hopkins, Peter Thielen and Tom Mehoke had spent years sequencing the genome of influenza. They were naturals to examine the work of the Chinese scientists as this new strain of coronavirus spread across the globe,. These biologists y are now using their experience from the Johns Hopkins' Applied Physics Laboratory to better understand the virus that causes COVID-19.

With software and molecular biology approaches developed in part at their Applied Physics Laboratory, Thielen and Mehoke use a handheld DNA sequencer to conduct immediate on-site genome sequencing of SARS-CoV-2—the virus that causes COVID-19.

"This information allows us to track the evolution of the virus," Thielen said. "It gives us a sense of where the new cases coming into Baltimore could've originated, and insight into how long transmission may have occurred undetected. There are a lot of things we can glean from that."

The virus causing COVID-19, Thielen said, does not appear to be mutating as fast. "When this virus was first sequenced in China, that information was helpful in starting the process to develop a vaccine," Thielen explained. "What we're doing informs whether or not the virus is mutating away from that original sequence, and how quickly. Based on the mutation rate, early data indicates that this would likely be a single vaccine rather than one that needs to be updated each year, like the flu shot." In the near-term, the mutations inform how the virus is spreading.

The resulting genomic sequence data has shown that Chinese authorities rapidly detected the epidemic and that the number of COVID-19 cases increased quickly because of human to human transmission after a single introduction into the human population.

Andersen and collaborators at several other research institutions used this sequencing data to explore the origins and evolution of SARS-CoV-2 by focusing in on several tell-tale features of the virus.

Mutations, which have occurred in the creation of the various strains in 2021, can explain how long the virus may have gone undetected and the supposition that there are likely far more cases than diagnosed, and can advise on what measures to put in place (such as the social-distancing efforts and closings that had been ongoing nationwide by State officials.

The peskiest of all at this time in the fall 2022 is the omicron subvariant of COVID-19, BA.5. It has become one of the dominant strains of the virus in the U.S. It's the most easily spread strain to date and is able to evade immunity from COVID infection and vaccination.

If you've been exposed to someone with the virus or have COVID-19 symptoms and are waiting for a test or your results, the word is stay home and isolate from others.

Sequencing of the virus' genome is being performed by scientists all over the globe now as they work to trace the source of regional outbreaks. In northern California, for example, news reports suggest that genome sequencing had originally linked the Bay Area outbreak to the Grand Princess cruise ship, which linked back to the virus found in Washington State, which likely came from China. Amazing.

That's the type of insight—a DNA fingerprint, if you will—that Thielen and Mehoke will gain as more virus genomes are sequenced from the Baltimore and Washington, D.C., regions.

These two biologists along with other scientists analyzed the genetic template for spike proteins, armatures on the outside of the virus that it uses to grab and penetrate the outer walls of human and animal cells. More specifically, they focused on two important features of the spike protein: the receptor-binding domain (RBD), a kind of grappling hook that grips onto host cells, and the cleavage site, a molecular can opener that allows the virus to crack open and enter host cells.

For a layman, that explains it very well.

The scientists found that the RBD portion of the SARS-CoV-2 spike proteins had evolved to effectively target a molecular feature on the outside of human cells called ACE2, a receptor involved in regulating blood pressure. The SARS-CoV-2 spike protein was so effective at binding the human cells, in fact, that the scientists concluded it was the result of natural selection and not the product of genetic engineering. Evidence to the contrary now shows it was manufactured.

It took a while for this to be the prevalent conclusion as for a long time, it seemed that the conclude was that the virus is the product of natural evolution." The speculation today is that it was brought about by deliberate function-gain genetic engineering."

SARS-CoV-2 could have evolved such a virulent cleavage site in human cells and soon kicked off the current epidemic, as the coronavirus would possibly have become far more capable of spreading between people.

Study co-author Andrew Rambaut cautioned that it was difficult if not impossible to know early on which of the scenarios is most likely. If the SARS-CoV-2 entered humans in its current pathogenic form from an animal source, it raises the probability of future outbreaks, as the illness-causing strain of the virus could still be circulating in the animal population and might once again jump into humans.

The chances are lower of a non-pathogenic coronavirus entering the human population and then evolving properties similar to SARS-CoV-2.

Funding for the research was provided by the US National Institutes of Health, the Pew Charitable Trusts, the Wellcome Trust, the European Research Council, and an ARC Australian Laureate Fellowship.

For a non-scientist and a non-biologist such as myself, I am glad there is no test on the information above. It pleases me to no end, however, that there are such brilliant people with such great knowledge to study and dissect the makeup of this current pandemic. They not only pass these tough tests every day, they construct tests so that others can learn from their work.

They are working to make our world a safer place to live and to create the biological armaments to fight and defeat diseases and viruses such as those associated with Covid-19.

CHAPTER 3

The Virus Remedy Across the World!

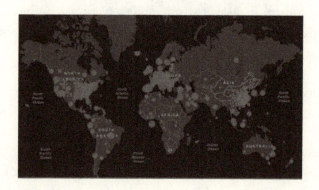

Why did it happen? Why was the world response so inept? Why did so many people die? Has washing hands and avoiding neighbors ever solved a pandemic in our past?

The whole world did not completely go in total lockdown but from those of us living through this nightmare, no matter in which country we live, it sure seems total.

As of today, there are 210 countries and territories that are affected by the coronavirus. It is worthy of note that Sub-Sahara Africa's numbers of cases and deaths are substantially less than most countries which have the virus.

Why? Because the areas discussed are mosquito malaria prone. The people who live there, if they are living, after DDT was banned have already been treated with chloroquine or hydroxychloroquine for years to prevent and to cure their malaria in this area of the world. It seems to have worked.

Too bad some of the great scientific minds do not see this as a relevant piece of data that hydroxychloroquine does help substantially in the treatment of COVID-10

For many years US travelers have taken prophylactic shots (small dosages with effects lasting several or more weeks) to not get malaria while they hunted big game in Africa. If the big game had its way, it would have banned both chloroquine and hydroxychloroquine. Meanwhile, since the evidence of a COVID-19 cure is only anecdotal, the rest of the world is struggling more so and dying with the pandemic.

The story of this nasty bug as noted in prior chapters shows that it first surfaced in the Chinese seafood and poultry market late in the year two-years ago, and migrated through human transfer to the 210 assorted countries killing many and sickening more than one and a million in just a matter of weeks. The World Health Organization wasted no time declaring the situation a pandemic.

As a result of the penetration and spread of the virus, almost all countries instituted a number of remedies to mitigate the virus.

Almost simultaneously, countries adopted similar approaches to keep from contracting this deadly virus. Still the officials suggest that limiting face-to-face contact with others is the best way to reduce the spread of coronavirus disease 2019 aka (COVID-19). Besides quarantine, a major recommendation is to wash hands frequently with soap and water or hand sanitizers and practice a technique that has been dubbed as social distancing.

Social distancing is also called "physical distancing." It is a self-described term in many ways meaning *keeping space between yourself and other people outside of your home.* To practice social or physical distancing, here are some basic rules:

- Stay at least 6 feet (2 meters) from other people.
- Science says three feet is adequate.
- Do not gather in groups.
- Stay out of crowded places and avoid mass gatherings.

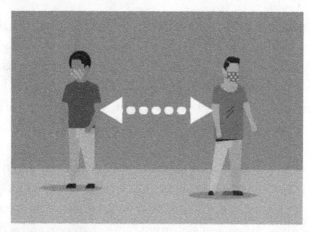

Picture is worth a thousand words What is social distancing?

In addition to everyday steps to prevent COVID-19, keeping space between you and others is one of the best tools we have to avoid being exposed to this virus and slowing its spread locally and across the country and world. Since there are no recommended therapeutics other than the anecdotal evidence reported by doctors who have great success using hydroxychloroquine with their COVID-19 patients and of course there are the three vaccines introduced late 2020 and highly available in 2021--(Moderna, Pfizer, Johnson & Johnson) for the COVID-19 disease.

The objective of most people is to not get it. When the infection comes to town, stay away from other humans who do not live in your immediate residence. With the other strains, it is wise to keep your distance from even the known vaccinated.

Here are some other recommendations:

When COVID-19 is spreading in your area, everyone should limit close contact with individuals outside your household in indoor and outdoor spaces. Since people can spread the virus before they know they are sick, it is important to stay away from others when possible, even if you have no symptoms. Social distancing is especially important for people who are at higher risk of getting very sick – those with other health issues and those over 65-years of age. Unless you are using an N-95 mask, most masks are ineffective as the disease is smaller than the holes in the mask material.

Why should I practice social distancing?

COVID-19 spreads mainly among people who are in close contact (within about 3-6 feet) for a prolonged period. Spread happens when an infected person coughs, sneezes, or talks, and droplets from their mouth or nose are launched into the air and land in the mouths or noses or eyes of people nearby. Just because you don't see it happening, does not mean it is not happening. Imagine that everybody you speak with or come closer than 3-6 feet or so to you is spreading these contagious droplets and this makes you even safer. Think about avoiding the disease.

But if you get this disease, make sure you are comfortable with the recommended treatment. Make sure your doctor is not politically motivated. Keep your family apprised of what you feel is best. For me, it would be hydroxychloroquine as the proper therapeutic because, well, quite frankly it is because I think the bogus testing of hydroxychloroquine in test cases has proven nothing other than how political medical science has become.

The droplets can infect just by being in the opening passages of your airways but can also be inhaled into the lungs. Recent studies indicate that people who are infected but do not have symptoms likely also play a role in the spread of COVID-19.

You can also get the COVID-19 virus by touching a surface or object that has the virus on it and then touching your own mouth, nose, or eyes. This is a minor way of spreading the disease but avoid having the issue by keeping surfaces sanitized. However, again, this is not thought to be the main way the virus spreads. COVID-19 can live for hours or days on a surface, depending on factors such as sun light and humidity. Social distancing helps limit contact with infected people and contaminated surfaces. Stay away from where the infection is known to be.

Although the risk of severe illness may be different for everyone, anyone can get and spread COVID-19. Everyone has a role to play in slowing the spread and protecting themselves, their family, and their community. For some people, the risk of not paying attention to social distancing can be to suffer death after a long illness with the virus.

Here are some tips for social distancing especially when the disease is spreading.

- Follow guidance from authorities where you live.
- If you need to shop for food or medicine at the grocery store or pharmacy, stay at least 3-6 feet away from others.
- Use mail-order for medications, if possible.
- Consider a grocery delivery service.
- Cover your mouth and nose with a cloth face cover when around others, including when you have to go out in public, for example

to the grocery store. There is no 100% mask but N-95s so far are rated best.
- Stay at least 3-66 feet between yourself and others, even when you wear a face covering.
- Avoid large and small gatherings in private places and public spaces, such a friend's house, parks, restaurants, shops, or any other place. It is safer outdoors for sure. This advice applies to people of any age, including teens and younger adults. Children should not have in-person playdates while school is out. To help maintain social connections while social distancing, learn tips to keep children healthy while school is out. Keep up to date with the news on COVID and speak to a doctor you trust.
- Work from home when possible.
- If possible, avoid using any kind of public transportation, ridesharing, or taxis.
- If you are a student or parent, talk to your school about options for digital/distance learning.

Stay connected while staying away.

It is very important to stay in touch with friends and family that don't live in your home. Call, video chat, or stay connected using social media. Everyone reacts differently to stressful situations and having to socially distance yourself from someone you love can be difficult. Read tips for stress and coping.

What is the difference between quarantine and isolation?

We have heard there is some concern out there about the differences between isolation and quarantine. The following should help in their differentiation:

Quarantine

Quarantine is used to **keep someone who** might **have been exposed to COVID-19 away from others.** Someone in self-quarantine decides on their own to stay separated from others, and they limit movement outside of their home or current place. A person may have been exposed to the virus without knowing it (for example, when traveling or out in the community), or they could have the virus without feeling symptoms. Quarantine helps limit further spread of COVID-19.

Isolation

Isolation is used to **separate sick people from healthy people**. People who are in isolation should stay home. In the home, anyone sick should separate themselves from others by staying in a specific "sick" bedroom or space and using a different bathroom (if possible). It is not a good idea as was done in NY, NJ, PA, and Michigan to take recovering COVID patients and mix them with a healthy nursing home population.

What should I do if I might have been exposed? If I feel sick? Or have confirmed COVID-19?

All people should self-monitor all the time.

When monitoring yourself, be alert for symptoms; do the following

- Watch for fever,* cough, or shortness of breath.
- Take your temperature if symptoms develop.
- Practice social distancing. Maintain 6 feet of distance from others, and stay out of crowded places.
- Contact a physician if you believe you have symptoms.
- Make sure you get a good therapeutic. I think Hydroxychloroquine, zinc, vitamin D, A, and a good zinc enabler is a very good choice but I am not a doctor. r

What do I mean by a zinc enabler. First of all remember that Zinc needs a little help to do its job.

Studies show that zinc can block the replication and growth of viruses in the body and in lab tests. In the body, zinc improves the actions of immune cells like Neutrophils, T cells, B cells and NK that act as the police of the body, which attack infections.

The search for a natural option for reducing viral load. Zinc is found and operates in every cell of the body, but it's a non-fat-soluble mineral that can't move through the fat-based cell membrane. Therefore, it needs help to cross the cell membrane from special transport systems. These systems include zinc ionophore and zinc binding-proteins. The zinc binding-proteins are located in all membranes of every cell of the body for efficient inflow and outflow of zinc in the cells. Red wine has small amounts of what is needed. So make sure you don't depend just on red wine.

What should you do if you feel healthy but: you recently had close contact with a person with COVID-19, or you recently traveled from somewhere outside the U.S. or you just came from a cruise ship or river boat

- Self-Monitor
- Self-Quarantine
- Check your temperature twice a day and watch for symptoms.
- Stay home for 14 days and self-monitor.
- If possible, stay away from people who are high-risk for getting very sick from COVID-19.

If you feel healthy but have been diagnosed with COVID-19, or Are waiting for test results, or have symptoms such as cough, fever, or shortness of breath

- Self-Isolate
- Stay in a specific sick room or area and away from other people.
- If possible, use a separate bathroom.

- Read as much important information about caring for yourself or someone else who is sick.

Look up such important information on the Internet or ask your family doctor about:

- How to Protect Yourself
    - Social Distancing
    - Face Mask
- Cleaning and Disinfecting Your Home
    - Lysol
    - Wash hands with soap & water
- Gatherings and Community Events
    - Social Distancing
    - Masks

CHAPTER 4

The World Declared a Lockdown!

The reference document for parts of this chapter was written by Derrick Bryson Taylor for the New York Times on April 7, 2020. Much of the information on the COVID remains the same over time. Thank you Derrick for the fine job.

As you can see from the map of restrictions, the whole world was not completely in total lockdown but from those of us living through this nightmare, no matter in which country we live, it sure seems like it was. The below chart has gotten better and gotten worse as countries learned about the virus and either toughened restrictions or loosened them to suit the needs of their country.

RESTRICTIONS IN PLACE	SCHOOLS	PUBS AND BARS	SPORTING EVENTS	MASS GATHERINGS	TRAVEL RESTRICTIONS
UK		•	•	•	•
GERMANY	•			•	•
USA	•		•	•	•
PORTUGAL	•	•	•	•	•
SPAIN	•	•	•	•	•
IRELAND	•	•	•	•	
DENMARK	•		•	•	•
SWITZERLAND	•	•	•	•	•
FRANCE	•	•	•	•	
BELGIUM	•	•		•	
NORWAY	•	•	•	•	•
MALTA	•	•	•	•	•
ISRAEL	•	•	•	•	•
ITALY	•	•	•	•	•

As of the date of this report, there were 195 countries (210 countries and territories) that were affected by the coronavirus. As discussed earlier in this book, and I repeat below because it is important, it is worthy of note that Sub-Sahara Africa's numbers of cases and deaths are substantially less than most countries which have the virus. Why? Speculation is that the areas are mosquito malaria prone. That would mean that the people have been treated with chloroquine and hydroxychloroquine for years to prevent and to cure malaria in this area of the world. These two drugs are reported to have a prophylactic (preventative) effect on the Corona virus also. Meanwhile the rest of the world is struggling more so with the pandemic.

The story of this nasty bug as noted in prior chapters shows that it first surfaced in the Chinese seafood and poultry market late last year, and migrated through human transfer to the 210 assorted countries killing many and sickening more than one and a half million in just a matter of weeks. The World Health Organization wasted no time declaring the situation a pandemic.

We will discuss potential cures and the politics behind such cures in later chapters. For now, let's explore the lockdowns.

There were many unforeseen and unpredicted impacts of the COVID-19 pandemic lockdown across the globe. As the global lockdown in most countries has recently been lifted but in a phased manner, it still is a good idea to explore its impacts to understand its consequences comprehensively. Theoretically of this science is accepted more than the true science of COVID, it can guide future decisions that will be made in a possible future wave of the COVID-19 pandemic or other global disease outbreak. The future is the future.

At first to most people who never faced a pandemic before, the lockdowns and mandates appeared logical and were met by the public as members of the team. So, at first, there appeared to be an improved capacity to manage the disease and that lockdown and other contrived ad hoc measures employed in its control at least seemed to be effective with all the positive hype to do something.

The global lockdown was a unique phenomenon prompted by the desire to protect lives from the ravaging pandemic. It was adopted on two fronts, namely, domestic and international. Domestically, the government restricted people's movement and instructed confinement to homes, thus limiting if not entirely halting the daily interactions between humans.

On the other hand, countries locked down national borders, restricting the movement of people and goods thus hampering the economic and human relations that had previously existed among countries. It did not take long for people across the world to begin to resist lockdowns and other authoritative measures to control the populations.

The global lockdown also affected how people access food, disrupting the production of certain food products. Overall, the global agricultural market remained stable although with some increase in the production of food staples such as rice, wheat and maize.

The lockdown which resulted in many people out of work impacted the global economy. Of course. This should not have come as a surprise. Many countries' restrictive measures including the measures in many of the states in the US resulted in issues that had been given little thought before implementation.

At first everybody seemed OK to deal with these measures since we were all on the same team but later, we realized that in many cases, the cure was worse than the disease.

The closure of schools, for example had multiple and varying effects on young people as they experience a disruption in their education. There was a major issue caused by the impact of the global lockdown on tourism, hospitality, sports, and leisure. People really were getting agitated and it is no wonder things were able to be kept without a revolution.

The fact is that with the onset of the COVID-19 pandemic lockdowns, there were high profile lay-offs, bankruptcies and request for business and personal aid, even amongst the airlines which saw a massive decline in patronage. The global lockdown fundamentally altered the everyday life of individuals across the globe, mostly in a negative way. President Biden was ruthless in his insistence on lockdowns and mandated and he hurt the military in his response to COVID.

Not just the military but that impact was especially noticeable as heroes were published for not being vaccinated. Millions and millions of Americans have had their lives impacted by President Joe Biden's COVID-19 vaccine mandates. Whether you happen to drive a truck, work in health care or as noted, serve in the armed forces, your job more than likely was threatened by the Biden administration.

The coercive approach put Washington in charge of making very personal health decisions. The message from the Biden Administration was very clear: If you don't follow the mandate, you could lose your job or your employer will be severely fined. Thankfully the Supreme Court struck down the Occupational Safety and Health Administration mandate, providing much needed relief for employers, employees and families across Michigan.

Sadly, as noted, one area that hasn't gotten enough attention as it should is the mandate's impact on our servicemen and women. When Biden made the decision to mandate COVID-19 vaccinations for members of the military, his administration began to dishonorably discharge those who did not want the vaccine. This was altered somewhat because it would have negatively impacted future opportunities for the men and women serving our nation who refused the vaccine.

Very few Americans felt that these men and women should have been discharged at all for exercising their religious or medical freedom.

It is not a small number of soldiers who refused to take the vaccine. As of Jan. 26, the Army reported that 3,350 soldiers had refused the jab. No military person could believe they would be fired.

Nobody is sure of the long-term impact or the magnitude of the COVID-19 pandemic and the attendant global lockdown impacts. However, as events unfold, what has been observed is the rapid decline in social interactions, a looming global economic depression, loss of lives, and the growing fear of the 'unknown' and consequently the alteration of the status quo. Furthermore, the COVID-19 pandemic has had far-reaching effects on the world, including a huge burden on the healthcare systems of different nations, mortalities and other diseases/health challenges.

Apart from the health-related effects of the COVID-19, there are other impacts of the consequent lockdown, which has affected the globe, which this review has outlined across various strata of life. There have been scrambles to obtain proper treatments and strategies to manage the pandemic to quickly ease the world back to normal, including several drug and vaccines, studies to understand the epidemiology of the disease and effects on ageing. While these are ongoing, a broader socioeconomic strategy needs to be developed to mitigate the pandemic's negative impacts.

Sustainable business models need to be developed along with food security and long-term plans to stabilize the global economy while guarding it against the risks of recession which hovers in the future as these are not the most robust times with Biden's self-induced energy crisis and inflation.

Even Biden is confused about whether the pandemic is still in play. He is likely confused by the ever-changing nature of the global pandemic, variations in the levels of lockdown amongst different countries and even levels of lockdown implementation. As noted, the effects associated with the lockdown cut across all countries of the world and still require focused and dedicated efforts for their mitigation. We have a long road to travel to make this all right.

Discounting real solutions such as Hydroxychloroquine and Ivermectin for political reasons is certainly not our best strategy for the future.

CHAPTER 5

History of COVID-19—What Happened When?

I can show a fairly accurate timeline of the outbreak so far that may help put the origination and some destinations of this coronavirus in perspective. This timeline takes us to about a year ago If I continued the timeline, a lot of what would be shown would be repeats as not much work has been done that tilts the Hydroxychloroquine and Ivermectin scales one bit.

We have learned that the virus itself was brewing in November 2019 and perhaps even before that.

17 November 17, 2019
There is a report from by the South China Morning Post (SCMP) on 13 March 2020, that a 55-year-old man who was later confirmed with the novel coronavirus, may have contracted the disease on 17 November 2019. This apparently is the best information so far about the earliest date of virus contraction.

Dec 1, 2019
The earliest traceable and confirmed patient, the 55-year-old man started experiencing symptoms on 1 December 2019. According to the

report, he had not been to the Huanan Seafood Wholesale Market of Wuhan. No epidemiological link could be found between this case and later cases. This is not confirmed

Dec 2, 2019]
A 51-year-old Dongguan doctor suddenly developed a cough and fever and was hospitalized. This is the first known hospitalization caused by the pneumonia with unknown causes. The patient had a lung infection, severe pneumonia, acute respiratory distress syndrome, and allergic purpura. No epidemiological link could be found between this case and later cases. As of mid-January 2020, his diagnosis included Streptococcus pneumoniae and fungi. The tests for COVID-19 had been developed only days before this report.

Dec 10, 2019
Before the determinations on earlier cases, there was a 57-year-old seafood merchant working at the Huanan Seafood Wholesale Market. He is considered by some to be the first patient< The source for this is a March 6, 2020 report by The Wall Street Journal. As you can see, this early information is sketchy at best.

Dec 12, 2019
On January 9, 2020, the Thai online news Thaiger reported the new viral outbreak was first detected in the city of Wuhan on 12 December 2019. The source of this information was not provided in the news report.

Dec 16, 2019
The patient known as first traceable patient, the 55-year-old man, was admitted to Wuhan Central Hospital with infection in both lungs. He was resistant to anti-flu drugs.

Dec 20–29, 2019
During this period, members of the Wuhan Institute of Virology and others reported and published a report on seven cases of people with

severe pneumonia who were admitted to the intensive care unit of the Wuhan Jin Yin-Tan Hospital at the beginning of the outbreak. A patient labeled as ICU-01 was not proven to be linked to the Wuhan Seafood Market, but the other six were either sellers or deliverymen at the market. Speculation was that the live market would play a major role in the determination of the cause.

Dec 21, 2019
Chinese epidemiologists published in the CCDC Weekly (Chinese Center for Disease Control and Prevention) Jan 21, 2020 edition, an article stating that their first cluster of patients with "pneumonia of an unknown cause" occurred beginning on Dec 21, 2019.

Dec 24, 2019
Doctors from the Central Hospital of Wuhan took fluid samples from the lungs of a 65-year-old deliveryman who worked at the Wuhan seafood market and sent them to Vision Medicals, Guangzhou, for further testing.

Dec 25, 2019
China's Youth Daily, Wuhan Fifth Hospital gastroenterology director Lu Xiaohong said that she heard that some of the hospital staff might be infected by this unknown agent on Dec 25.

Dec 26-27
Zhang Jixian, the Director of the Department of Respiratory and Critical Care at Hubei Provincial Hospital of Integrated Chinese & Western Medicine, examined an elderly couple who presented themselves at the hospital with fever and cough on Dec 26, 2019. CT scans of their chests showed a different pattern from other viral pneumonias. She asked the couple's son to undergo a scan and found the same pattern. But, he had showed symptoms. Another patient, who was employed as a merchant from the Huanan Seafood Wholesale Market, arrived at the hospital with a fever and cough that same day. After conducting normal tests, Zhang ruled out known respiratory ailments. She reportedly believed

this was an infectious disease. She reported the four cases to her superiors at the hospital on Dec 27, 2019..

Vision Medicals had sequenced most of the virus from fluid samples of the 65-year-old deliveryman sent by Central Hospital of Wuhan on Dec 27. The results showed an alarming similarity to the deadly SARS coronavirus that was prevalent between 2002 and 2003.

Dec 28-29, 2019
During the following two days, three similar cases were received by the Hubei Provincial. They were all associated with the seafood market. On Dec 29, the hospital administration convened a multi-departmental panel of doctors. The doctors concluded that the cases were unusual and required special attention. They thus reported their findings to the provincial CDC.

Wuhan CDC staff initiated a field investigation and found additional patients with similar symptoms who were linked to the market. This is attributed to a CCDC publication—the initial admissions to Hubei Provincial Hospital occurred on Dec 29

Dec 30, 2019
There was a genetic sequencing report from CapitalBio Medlab of Beijing about the pathogen of a 41 year-old-patient, the sample of which was collected by Wuhan Central Hospital mistakenly diagnosed as Severe acute respiratory syndrome coronavirus (SARS coronavirus). This mistaken result alerted the authority and some of the Wuhan doctors of the issue.

Wuhan Municipal Health Committee issued an "urgent notice on the appropriate treatment to patients with pneumonia of unknown cause" to medical institutions under its jurisdiction.

Multiple doctors in Wuhan examined and shared the test report via the internet, including Li Wenliang, an ophthalmologist at Wuhan Central

Hospital. Li posted a warning to alumni from his medical school class via a WeChat group in the late afternoon that a cluster of seven patients treating within the ophthalmology department had been unsuccessfully treated for symptoms of viral pneumonia and diagnosed with SARS. These patients did not respond to traditional treatments, and so they were quarantined in an ER department of the Wuhan Central Hospital.

In the WeChat post, Li posted the erroneous diagnostics that "there had been 7 confirmed cases of SARS". Li posted a snippet of an RNA analysis finding "SARS coronavirus" and extensive bacteria colonies in a patient's airways. Thereafter, news of an outbreak of "pneumonia of unknown origin" started circulating on social media on the evening of Dec 30, 2019.

Dec 31, 2019
This is where the World Health Organization gets involved. The Wuhan Municipal Health Committee informed WHO that 27 "cases of pneumonia of unknown etiology (unknown cause) were detected in Wuhan." Most worked in the stalls at the Huanan Seafood Wholesale Market, seven of whom by this time, were in critical condition.

Chinese state television CCTV ch13 in their daily news broadcasts issued an epidemiological alert telling entire country of a strange and unknown virus found. It also reported that a team of experts from the National Health Commission had arrived in Wuhan on the day to lead the investigation. The People's Daily said the exact cause remained unclear and it would be premature to speculate."

A vendor at the Huanan Seafood Market, named Qu Shiqian said that government officials had disinfected the market premises on Dec 31, 2019 and told stallholders (those who worked in the market stalls) to wear face masks. Qu said he had only learned of the pneumonia outbreak from media reports. "Previously I thought they had flu," he said. "It should be not serious. We are fish traders. How can we get infected?"

Tao Lina, a public health expert and former official with Shanghai's Centre for disease control and prevention, said, "I think we are [now] quite capable of killing it in the beginning phase, given China's disease control system, emergency handling capacity and clinical medicine support." No human-to-human infection had been reported so far and more pathological tests and investigations were underway, official said.

As a result of the official announcement of the Wuhan Municipal Health Commission, Hong Kong, Macau and Taiwan immediately tightened their inbound screening processes Hong Kong Secretary for Food and Health Sophia Chan Siu-chee announced after an urgent night-time meeting with officials and experts, "[any suspected cases] including the presentation of fever and acute respiratory illness or pneumonia, and travel history to Wuhan within 14 days before onset of symptoms, we will put the patients in isolation.".

The social media reports stated that 27 patients in Wuhan—most of them stallholders at the Huanan Seafood Market—had been treated for the mystery illness.

On the Financial Times of March 20, 2020, they stated "Taiwan said its doctors had heard from mainland colleagues that medical staff were getting ill — a sign of human-to-human transmission. Taipei officials said they reported this to both International Health Regulations (IHR), a WHO framework for exchange of epidemic prevention and response data between 196 countries, and Chinese health authorities on December 31."

Dec 31, 2019
Chinese authorities treated dozens of cases of pneumonia of unknown cause. The government in Wuhan, China, confirmed that health authorities were treating dozens of cases. Days later, researchers in China identified a new virus that had infected dozens of people in Asia.

Jan 11, 2020

China reported its first death. On Jan. 11, Chinese state media reported the first known death from an illness caused by the virus, which had infected dozens of people. The 61-year-old man who died was a regular customer at the market in Wuhan, and he had previously been found to have abdominal tumors and chronic liver disease. The report of his death came just before one of China's biggest holidays, when hundreds of millions of people travel across the country.

Jan 20, 2020

Other countries, including the United States, began to confirm cases. The first confirmed cases outside mainland China occurred in Japan, South Korea and Thailand, according to the World Health Organization's first situation report. The first confirmed case in the United States came the next day in Washington State, where a man in his 30s developed symptoms after returning from a trip to Wuhan.

Jan 23, 2020

Wuhan is a city of more than 11 million people. It was abruptly cut off by the Chinese authorities.

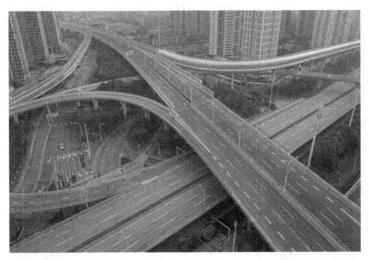

Chinese authorities suspended buses, subways and ferries within the city of Wuhan, pictured above on Feb. 3.Credit...Getty Images

The Chinese authorities closed off Wuhan by canceling planes and trains leaving the city, and suspending buses, subways and ferries within it. At this point, at least 17 people had died and more than 570 others had been infected, including in Taiwan, Japan, Thailand, South Korea and the United States.

Jan 30, 2020
W.H.O. then declared a global health emergency. Amid thousands of new cases in China, a "public health emergency of international concern" was officially declared by the W.H.O. China's Foreign Ministry spokeswoman said that it would continue to work with the W.H.O. and other countries to protect public health, and the U.S. State Department warned travelers to avoid China.

Jan 31, 2020
The Trump administration against the advice of mostly everybody decided that for the safety of Americans he would restrict travel from China. They suspended entry into the United States by any foreign national who had traveled to China in the past 14 days, excluding the immediate family members of American citizens or permanent residents. By this date, 213 people had died and nearly 9,800 had been infected worldwide.

Feb 2, 2020,
The first coronavirus death was reported outside China. A 44-year-old man in the Philippines died after being infected, officials said,. It was the first death reported outside China. By this point, more than 360 people had died.

Feb 5, 2020
A cruise ship in Japan, The Diamond Princess, a part of Princess Cruise Lines, quarantined thousands.

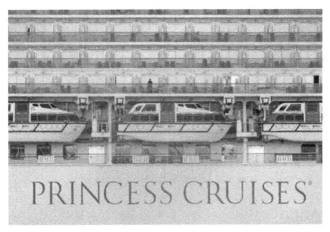

The Diamond Princess cruise ship on Feb. 9Credit...
Eugene Hoshiko/Associated Press

After a two-week trip to Southeast Asia, more than 3,600 passengers began a quarantine aboard the Diamond Princess cruise ship in Yokohama, Japan. Officials started screening passengers, and the number of people who tested positive became the largest number of coronavirus cases outside China. By Feb. 13, the number stood at 218.

Feb 7, 2020
A Chinese doctor who tried to raise the alarm died.

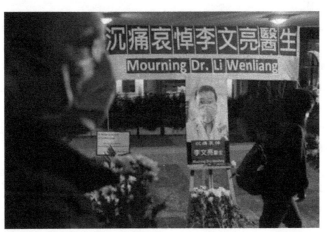

The death of Dr. Li Wenliang provoked anger at how the Chinese government handled the epidemic. Credit...Tyrone Siu/Reuters

When Dr. Li Wenliang, a Chinese doctor, died on Feb. 7 after contracting the coronavirus, he was hailed as a hero by many for trying to ring early alarms that a cluster of infections could spin out of control.

In early January, the authorities had reprimanded him, and he was forced to sign a statement denouncing his warning as an unfounded and illegal rumor. Dr. Li's death provoked anger and frustration at how the Chinese government mishandled the situation by not sharing information earlier and silencing whistle-blowers.

Feb 11, 2020
The disease which the virus causes got a new name. The World Health Organization on Feb. 11 proposed an official name for the disease the virus coronavirus causes: *Covid-19*, an acronym that stands for coronavirus disease 2019. The name makes no reference to any of the people, places, or animals associated with the coronavirus, given the Chinese goal to avoid a stigma of association.

By the next day, the death toll in China had reached 1,113 and the total number of confirmed cases rose to 44,653. There were 393 cases outside of China, in 24 countries at the time.

Feb 13, 2020
In China, there were more than 14,000 new cases in Hubei Province.

Officials added more than 14,840 new cases to the total number of infected in Hubei Province, and the ruling Communist Party ousted top officials there. The new cases set a daily record, coming after officials in Hubei seemed to be including infections that were diagnosed by using lung scans of symptomatic patients.

Feb 14, 2020
France announced the first coronavirus death in Europe.

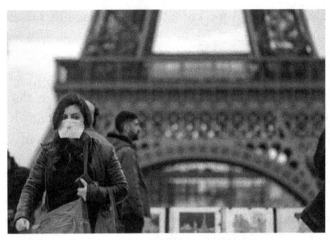

France's first coronavirus death was the fourth death from the virus outside of mainland China.
Credit...Ian Langsdon/EPA, via Shutterstock

An 80-year-old Chinese tourist died on Feb. 14 at a hospital in Paris, in what was the first coronavirus death outside Asia, the authorities said. It was the fourth death from the virus outside mainland China, where about 1,500 people had died, most of them in Hubei Province.

Feb 17, 2020
Chinese officials drafted legislation to curb the practice of eating wildlife such as that found in the aforementioned market. China said it was reviewing its trade and consumption of wildlife, which has been identified as a probable source of the outbreak. Officials drafted legislation that aims to end "the pernicious habit of eating wildlife," a statement from the Standing Committee of the Congress said.

Feb 19, 2020
Hundreds are released from the quarantined cruise ship. After a two-week quarantine, 443 passengers began to leave the Diamond Princess cruise ship. It was the first day of an operation taking three days to offload people who tested negative for the virus and did not have symptoms. Passengers who shared cabins with infected patients

remained on the ship. A total of 621 people, including passengers and crew aboard the ship had been infected.

Feb 21, 2020
An outbreak in South Korea is linked to a secretive church. The Shincheonji Church of Jesus, a secretive church in South Korea was linked to a surge of infections in the country. The number of confirmed cases in the country rose above 200, and more than 400 other church members reported potential symptoms, health officials said.

As a result, the government shut down thousands of kindergartens, nursing homes and community centers, and put a stop to political rallies in the capital, Seoul.

Feb 21, 2020
The virus from an undetermined source infected people in Iran. On Feb. 19, Iran announced two coronavirus cases in the country, then hours later said that both patients had died. Two days later, the country announced two additional deaths. The source of the virus in Iran is unknown. By Feb. 20, the number of global cases had risen to nearly 76,000, according to the W.H.O.

Feb 23, 2020
Italy, which has a major trading relationship with China and which had many recent visits from Wuhan was affected by a major surge in coronavirus cases. Italian Officials began to lock down towns.

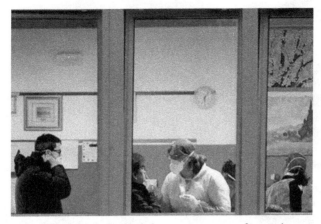

Officials in Italy locked down 10 towns after a cluster
of cases suddenly emerged near Milan.
Credit...Nicola Fossella/EPA, via Shutterstock

Europe faced its first major outbreak as the number of reported cases in Italy grew from fewer than five to more than 150. In the Lombardy region, officials locked down 10 towns after a cluster of cases suddenly emerged in Codogno, southeast of Milan. As a result, schools closed and sporting and cultural events were canceled.

Feb 24, 2020
The Trump administration began to get a feel for the enormity of this epidemic and asked Congress for $1.25 billion for a coronavirus response.

As the number of coronavirus cases around the globe continued to climb, the Trump administration began preparing for the virus to arrive in full scale in the United States. The White House asked Congress to allocate $1.25 billion in new emergency funds to bolster its preparedness — a significant escalation in the administration's response. At this point the United States, where Centers for Disease Control and Prevention officials warned of an almost certain outbreak, at this point, had 35 confirmed cases and no deaths.

Feb 24, 2020

Iran emerges as a second focus point of the virus.

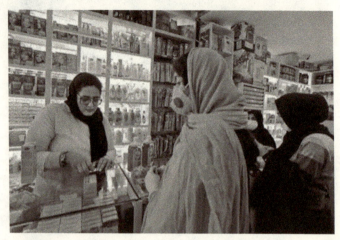

A number of other countries in the Middle East have reported coronavirus cases that have been linked back to Iran.
Credit...Atta Kenare/Agence France-Presse — Getty Images

At this point in the epidemic's spread, Iran said it had 61 coronavirus cases and 12 deaths, more than any other country but China, and public health experts warned that Iran was a cause for worry — its borders are crossed each year by millions of religious pilgrims, migrant workers and others. Cases in Iraq, Afghanistan, Bahrain, Kuwait, Oman, Lebanon, the United Arab Emirates and one in Canada, have been traced back to Iran. The US offered help to Iran but the offer was rejected.

Feb 26, 2020

Latin America reported its first coronavirus case. Brazilian health officials said that a 61-year-old São Paulo man, who had returned recently from a business trip to Italy, tested positive for the coronavirus. It was the first known case in Latin America. Officials also began tracking down other passengers on the flight the man took to Brazil and others who had contact with him in recent days.

Feb 28, 2020
The number of infections in Europe spikes. Italy, where 800 people had been infected by Feb. 28, remained an area of major concern. Cases in 14 other countries, including Northern Ireland and Wales, could be traced back to Italy. Germany had nearly 60 cases by Feb. 27, and France reported 57, more than triple the number from two days earlier. Both England and Switzerland reported additional cases, while Belarus, Estonia and Lithuania all reported their first infections.

Feb 28, 2020
Sub-Saharan Africa recorded its first infection.

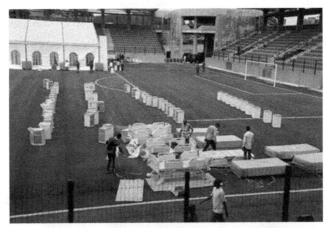

Nigeria's first confirmed case was an Italian
citizen returning to the country.
Credit...Pius Utomi Ekpei /Agence France-Presse — Getty Images

Nigeria, Africa's most populous nation, confirmed its first case of coronavirus on Feb. 28. The patient was an Italian citizen who had returned to Lagos from Milan.

Feb 29, 2020
The United States recorded its first coronavirus death and announced additional travel restrictions. The West Coast got some of the first infections seemingly because of many flights from China before the travel ban took place.

A patient near Seattle became the first coronavirus patient to die in the United States on Feb. 28. As the number of global cases rose to nearly 87,000, the Trump administration issued its highest-level warning, known as a "do not travel" warning, for areas in Italy and South Korea most affected by the virus. The government also banned all travel to Iran and barred entry to any foreign citizen who had visited Iran in the previous 14 days.

March 3, 2020
U.S. officials approve widespread coronavirus testing. The C.D.C. lifted all federal restrictions on testing for the coronavirus on March 3, according to Vice President Mike Pence. The news came after the C.D.C.'s first attempt to produce a diagnostic test kit fell flat. By this point, the coronavirus had infected more than 90,000 around the globe and killed about 3,000, according to the W.H.O.

March 11, 2020
President Trump restricted / blocked visitors from continental Europe.

In a prime-time address from the Oval Office, Mr. Trump said he would halt travelers from European countries other than Britain for 30 days, as the World Health Organization declared the coronavirus a pandemic and stock markets plunged further.

March 13, 2020
President Trump declares a national emergency.

Mr. Trump officially declared a national emergency, and said he was making $50 billion in federal funds available to states and territories to combat the coronavirus. He also said he would give hospitals and doctors more flexibility to respond to the virus, including making it easier to treat people remotely.

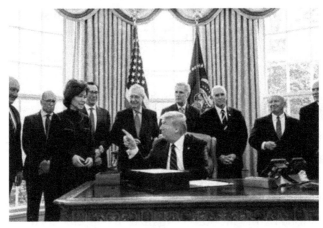

President Trump, who declared a national emergency, made millions of dollars in funds available to states.
Credit...Erin Schaff/The New York Times

March 15, 2020
The C.D.C. recommends no gatherings of 50 + people in the U.S.

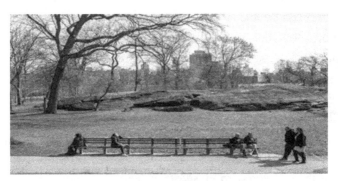

Central Park on March 18. President Trump advised citizens to avoid groups of more than 10.
Credit...Juan Arredondo for The New York Times

On March 15, the C.D.C. advised no gatherings of 50 or more people in the United States over the next eight weeks. The recommendation included weddings, festivals, parades, concerts, sporting events and conferences. The following day, Mr. Trump advised citizens to avoid groups of more than 10. New York City's public schools' system, the nation's largest with 1.1 million students, also announced that it would close.

March 16, 2020

Latin America begins to feel the effects of the virus. Several countries across Latin America imposed restrictions on their citizens to slow the spread of the virus. Venezuela announced a nationwide quarantine that began on March 17. Ecuador and Peru implemented countrywide lockdowns, while Colombia and Costa Rica closed their borders. However, Jair Bolsonaro, the president of Brazil, encouraged mass demonstrations by his supporters against his opponents in congress.

MARCH 17, 2020

France imposed a nationwide lockdown. On March 17, France imposed a nationwide lockdown, prohibiting gatherings of any size and postponing the second round its municipal elections. The lockdown was one of Europe's most stringent. While residents were told to stay home, officials allowed people to go out for fresh air but warned that meeting a friend on the street or in a park would be punishable with a fine. By this time, France had more than 6,500 infections with more than 140 deaths, according to the W.H.O.

MARCH 17

The E.U. barred most travelers from outside the bloc for 30 days.

European leaders voted to close off at least 26 countries to nearly all visitors from the rest of the world for at least 30 days. The ban on nonessential travel from outside the bloc was the first coordinated response to the epidemic by the European Union.

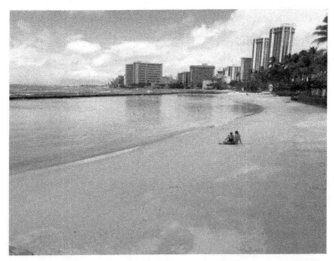

The European Union adopted a 30-day ban on non-essential travel to at least 26 European countries from the rest of the world.
Credit...Maria Contreras Coll for The New York Times

March 19, 2020

For the first time, China reported zero local infections. The report was specific: no new local infections for the previous day. This was a milestone in the ongoing fight against the pandemic. The news signaled that an end to China's epidemic could be in sight.

However, experts said the country would need to see at least 14 consecutive days without new infections for the outbreak to be considered over. And the announcement did not mean that China recorded no new coronavirus cases. Officials said that 34 new cases had been confirmed among people who had arrived in China from elsewhere.

March 21, 2020

Hospitals and other health care units were complaining that they did not have enough equipment to handle the volume of cases. Companies promised to begin to produce medical supplies to address the need. On March 21, the White House said that American companies were increasing efforts to restock hospitals with important supplies. Hanes and General Motors agreed to make masks and ventilators. Christian Siriano, a fashion designer, Dov Charney, the founder of Los Angeles Apparel, and Karla Colletto, a swimwear company, all agreed to repurpose their operations to create masks and hospital garments.

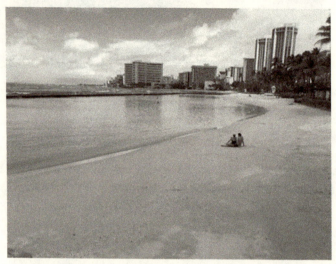

Gov. David Ige of Hawaii issued a mandatory two-week quarantine for anyone arriving in the state.
Credit...Caleb Jones/Associated Press

Hawaii's governor orders a mandatory 14-day quarantine to arriving visitors and residents. Gov. David Ige of Hawaii ordered a mandatory 14-day quarantine for everyone arriving in Hawaii, including tourists and returning residents. Mr. Ige called his order the first of its kind.

March 23, 2020
Prime Minister Boris Johnson locks Britain down.

The lockdown closed all nonessential shops, barred meetings of more than two people, and required all people to stay in their homes except for trips for food or medicine. Those who disobey risked being fined by the police.

March 24, 2020
Announcement: The Tokyo Olympics were delayed until 2021. Officials announced that the Summer Olympics in Tokyo would be postponed for one year. Only three previous Games had been canceled, all because of war: The 1916 Summer Olympics were canceled because of World War I, and the Summer and Winter Games were canceled in 1940 and 1944 because of World War II.

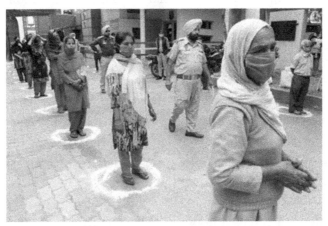

India ordered a three-week lockdown for its 1.3 billion citizens, and officials pledged to spend billions on medical supplies.
Credit...Narinder Nanu /Agence France-Presse — Getty Images

March 24, 2020
India, a country of 1.3 billion, announces a 21-day lockdown.

One day after the authorities halted all domestic flights, Narendra Modi, India's prime minister, declared a 21-day lockdown. While the number of reported cases in India was about 500, the prime minister pledged to spend about $2 billion on medical supplies, isolation rooms, ventilators and training for medical professionals.

March 26, 2020
The US eclipsed all other countries in confirmed coronavirus cases. The United States officially became the country hardest hit by the pandemic, with at least 81,321 confirmed infections and more than

1,000 deaths. This was more reported cases than in China, Italy or any other country.

March 27, 2020
President Trump signed the coronavirus stimulus bill into law. Mr. Trump signed a $2 trillion measure to respond to the coronavirus pandemic. Lawmakers said the bill, which passed with overwhelming support, was imperfect but essential to address the national public health and economic crisis.

March 28, 2020
The C.D.C. issued a travel advisory for the New York region. The C.D.C. urged residents of New York, New Jersey and Connecticut to "refrain from nonessential domestic travel for 14 days effective immediately." The advisory did not apply to workers in "critical infrastructure industries," including trucking, public health, financial services and food supply.

March 30, 2020
More states issue stay-at-home directives. Virginia, Maryland and Washington, D.C., issued orders requiring their residents to stay home. Similar orders went into effect for Kansas and North Carolina. Other states had previously put strict measures in place. The new orders meant that least 265 million Americans were being urged to stay home.

Apr 2, 2020
Global cases top 1 million, and millions loser their jobs. By April 2, the pandemic had sickened more than 1 million people in 171 countries across six continents, killing at least 51,000.

In just a few weeks, the pandemic put 22 million Americans out of work, including a staggering 6.6 million people who applied for unemployment benefits in the last week of March and another 5 million in the second week of April (22 million total). The speed and scale of the job losses was without precedent: Until March, the worst week for unemployment filings was 695,000 in 1982.

Apr 3, 2020
Health officials and government bureaucrats engage in debate over who should wear masks. The C.D.C unequivocally urged all Americans to wear a mask when they leave their homes. However, some officials called the recommendation voluntary and the President said that he had tested negative twice and did not see a need to wear one himself. "With the masks, it's going to be a voluntary thing," the president said. "You can do it. You don't have to do it. I am choosing not to do it. It may be good. It's only a recommendation, voluntary."

Apr 5, 2020
WH insiders continue to fight over therapeutic drug to fight coronavirus. There is no known cure for coronavirus. There is no vaccine and the scientists say the best hope is for a vaccine 18 months from now and that is unlikely. That would mean many, many more deaths.

Yet there is promise in a number of unofficial studies. Anthony Fauci calls these anecdotal meaning not proven by scientific trials, yet in the studies, patients are recovering. President Trump wants all Americans to have a right to try this drug and the evidence suggests he may be right, though he has no scientific proof, people are recovering.

Scoop: Inside the epic White House fight over hydroxychloroquine

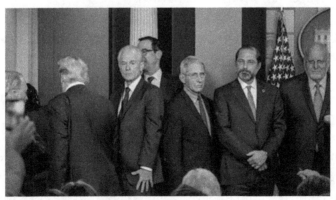

There is no peace at the Task Force Table
Photo: Drew Angerer /Getty Images

The White House coronavirus task force had its biggest fight yet on Saturday, pitting economic adviser Peter Navarro against infectious disease expert Anthony Fauci. At issue: How enthusiastically should the White House tout the prospects of an antimalarial drug to fight COVID-19?

Behind the scenes: This drama erupted into an epic Situation Room showdown. Trump's coronavirus task force gathered in the White House Situation Room on Saturday at about 1:30pm, according to four sources familiar with the conversation. Vice President Mike Pence sat at the head of the table.

Numerous government officials were at the table, including Fauci, coronavirus response coordinator Deborah Birx, Jared Kushner, acting Homeland Security Secretary Chad Wolf, and Commissioner of Food and Drugs Stephen Hahn.

Behind them sat staff, including Peter Navarro, tapped by Trump to compel private companies to meet the government's coronavirus needs under the Defense Production Act.

Toward the end of the meeting, Hahn began a discussion of the malaria drug hydroxychloroquine, which Trump believes could be a "game-changer" against the coronavirus.

Hahn gave an update about the drug and what he was seeing in different trials and real-world results.

Then Navarro got up. He brought over a stack of folders and dropped them on the table. People started passing them around.

"And the first words out of his mouth are that the studies that he's seen, I believe they're mostly overseas, show 'clear therapeutic efficacy,'" said a source familiar with the conversation. "Those are the exact words out of his mouth."

Navarro's comments set off a heated exchange about how the Trump administration and the president ought to talk about the malaria drug, which Fauci and other public health officials stress is unproven to combat COVID-19.

Fauci pushed back against Navarro, saying that there was only anecdotal evidence that hydroxychloroquine works against the coronavirus.

Researchers have said studies out of France and China are inadequate because they did not include control groups.

Fauci and others have said much more data is needed to prove that hydroxychloroquine is effective against the coronavirus.

As part of his role, Navarro has been trying to source hydroxychloroquine from around the world. He's also been trying to ensure that there are enough domestic production capabilities inside the U.S.

Fauci's mention of anecdotal evidence "just set Peter off," said one of the sources. Navarro pointed to the pile of folders on the desk, which included printouts of studies on hydroxychloroquine from around the world.

The reality is that people who were going to die are today still living and well. Anecdotal or not, people breathing to Navarro is more than enough proof.

April 6, 2020
Prime Minister Boris Johnson moved into intensive care after being admitted to the hospital with the virus. Ten days after going public with his coronavirus diagnosis, Prime Minister Boris Johnson of Britain was moved into intensive care. The decision was a precaution, according to the British government, who also said he had been in good spirits. Mr. Johnson had also asked the foreign secretary, Dominic Raab, to deputize for him "where necessary."

April 8, 2020
President Trump slammed the W.H.O. Over Coronavirus response and the truth. The president is not alone in his criticism

April 9, 2020
Prime Minister Boris Johnson has been moved out of intensive care but remains in hospital, Downing Street has said.

April 10, 2020
In today's briefing, the last which is included in this book, the confirmed cases of COVID-19 in the United States approach half a million, and the death toll has surpassed 16,500. But the speakers noted that there are pieces of promising news, including that the daily increase in new cases is leveling off and daily death tolls in hotspots like New York are also leveling off.

This is a signal that social distancing efforts undertaken weeks ago may actually be working. Surgeon General Jerome Adams, whose grave words comparing these weeks to 9/11 and Pearl Harbor, says that most of the U.S. won't be able to open by May 1 and when normal activities do resume it will be "place by place, bit by bit. We'll see.

There is that old Alka Seltzer ad that suggests "why trade a headache for an upset stomach." To some opening up the economy is necessary because the benefits of keeping it closed may disappear quickly if the when the economy is about to be resuscitated, it may be found that it has been dead too long! We'll see!

One thing is for sure if the hundreds of millions of hydroxychloroquine doses that have been acquired actually can prevent the disease as it seems it does and if it can cure the disease, then this makes opening the economy a lot less risky. 1. You can prevent getting it and 2. If you do get it, you can be cured for $20.00. The stakes are high

April summary:

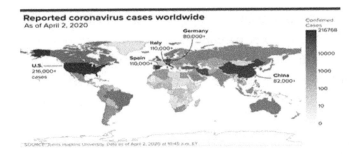

As cases continued to surge, countries keep their borders sealed. Businesses shut down (leading to massive job losses), schools close, sporting events cancel, and college students go home. People start wearing masks and practicing "social distancing."

May:

Experts focused on "flattening the curve," meaning that if you use a graph to map the number of COVID-19 cases over time, you would ideally start to see a flattened line representing a reduction of cases. After months in lockdown, states slowly begin a "phased reopening," based on criteria outlined by the Trump Administration, in coordination with state, county, and local officials. Meanwhile, scientists across the globe are in a race to understand the disease, find treatments and solutions, and develop vaccines.

The startling assets of the virus were in the early months. So, we modified the chart to simply recount monthly happenings instead of giving a daily toll.

June:

Efforts to reopen the economy leads to new cases, and the curve is not flattening. Experts point to the dangers of large gatherings and use terms like "clusters" and "super-spreader events."

July:

The pandemic is causing an uptick in mental health issues as job losses continue to soar, parents juggle working at home with caring for or homeschooling children, and young adults grow frustrated by isolation from friends and limited job prospects. Officials debate the best scenarios for allowing children to safely return to school in the fall.

August:

The first documented case of reinfection is reported in Hong Kong. On a broader scale, COVID-19 is now the third leading cause of death in the U.S. (after heart disease and cancer).

September:

The school year opened with a mix of plans to keep children and teachers safe, ranging from in-person classes to remote schooling to hybrid models. Meanwhile, the WHO recommends steroids to treat severely and critically ill patients, but not to those with mild disease. The Centers for Disease Control and Prevention (CDC) reports that people who had recently tested positive were about twice as likely to have reported dining at a restaurant than were those with negative test results.

October:

President Trump tests positive for COVID-19 after a gathering in the White House Rose Garden where multiple people were also thought to have been infected. Meanwhile, the Food and Drug Administration (FDA) grants full approval to a drug called remdesivir for treatment of COVID-19.

November:

Cases rise again as cold weather drives more people indoors—the U.S. begins to break records for daily cases/deaths. Many officials around the country bring plans for reopening to a halt. As the holidays approach, the CDC urges Americans to stay home, limit the size of their gatherings, and avoid mixing with people who don't live in their household.

December:

The FDA grants Pfizer-BioNTech the first Emergency Use Authorization (EUA) for an mRNA vaccine, a new type of vaccine that has proven to be highly effective against COVID-19. A week later, it grants another EUA to Moderna, also for an mRNA vaccine. But, as vaccinations begin, major variants of the virus are beginning to circulate. The UK reports that a new variant of the virus, called B.1.1.7, could be more contagious. By the end of the month, B.1.1.7 is detected in the U.S.

2021

January:

In the U.S., the number of cases and deaths begins to fall. But more variants are spreading, including one first identified in South Africa called B.1.351, which is reported in the U.S. by the end of the month. Around the world, the race is on to vaccinate as many people as possible in time to slow the spread of the variants. Researchers work to understand how deadly or contagious variants are compared to the original virus.

February:

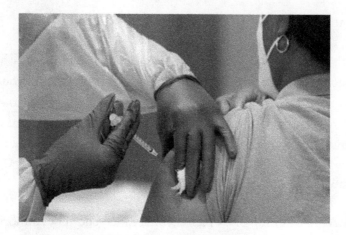

There is not enough vaccine supply to meet the demand. But the Biden Administration expects the addition of a third option (by Johnson & Johnson) to make vaccines more available to everyone. Meanwhile, companies are working to tweak their products to make distribution easier and to control new variants. So, while there may be hope that the end is in sight for the pandemic, it's highly probable that we will still be wearing masks and taking other precautions for some time to come.

March

On March 2, Texas and Mississippi announced that they would fully reopen, with Texas scheduling it on March 10 and Mississippi scheduling it on March 3. Both states continued to make recommendations but also they repealed all mandates. By March 5, more than 2,750 cases of COVID-19 variants were detected in 47 states; Washington, D.C.; and Puerto Rico. This number consisted of 2,672 cases of the B.1.1.7 variant, 68 cases of the B.1.351 variant, and 13 cases of the P.1 variant. On March 8, the U.S. passed 29 million cases. On March 11, President Joe Biden held his first prime time address of his presidency. In it, he announced his plan to push states to make vaccines available to all adults by May 1, with the aim to make small gatherings possible by the 4th of July. On March 24, the U.S. total cases passed 30 million, just as a number of states began to expand the eligibility age for COVID-19 vaccines. By March 27, more than 8,000 cases of the B.1.1.7 variant were reported across 51 jurisdictions.

]April

By April 1, more than 11,000 cases of the B.1.1.7 variant were reported, mostly in Florida and Michigan.]By April 7, the B.1.1.7 variant had become the dominant COVID-19 strain in America. On April 9, the # of U.S. cases passed 31 million. On April 12, six cases of a new "double mutant" SARS-CoV-2 variant from India were discovered (B.1.617) in California. On April 22, the U.S. total was over 32 million cases. On April 29, the CDC estimated that at least 35% of the U.S. population had been infected with the virus as of March 2021. That number was about four times higher than the official reported numbers. Not sure what that means. Was the lack of reporting intentional?

May

On May 6, a study by the Institute for Health Metrics and Evaluation found that the true COVID-19 death toll in the U.S. was more than 900,000 people. On May 13, the CDC changed its guidance and said that fully vaccinated individuals do not need to wear masks in most situations. On May 19, the U.S. total eclipsed 33 million cases.

June

On June 15, the U.S. # of deaths his 600,000.]

July

By July 7, the Delta variant was the most prevalent and the most worrisome. It had surpassed the Alpha variant to become the dominant COVID-19 strain in the U.S., according to CDC data. On July 17, the U.S. went past 34 million cases. On July 27, based on updated information for fully vaccinated people that new evidence on the Delta variant had provided, CDC added a recommendation for those people to wear a mask in public indoor settings in areas of substantial or high transmission. CDC also made other recommendations based on this information.[52]

August

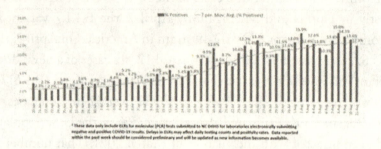

On August 1, 2021, the U.S. passed 35 million cases. On August 10, the U.S. passed 36 million cases. The number as we close out 2022 is up to 97 million cases. That's why most believe we have reached herd immunity. Though it has weakened the impact, it is still here. The prior timeline got us to a year from today.

CHAPTER 6

The "Cures"

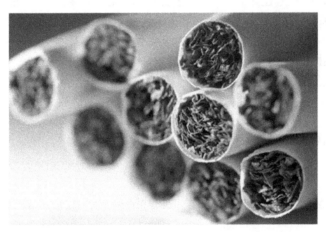

Could tobacco cure coronavirus? Don't laugh.

Though there is a lot of hope for a definitive cure for coronavirus, so far, no dice—officially at least. Even the Phizer and Moderna vaccinations did not pan out to be what we expected. A vaccination was to prevent diseases which they target. This did not happen though it is claimed that they lessened the impact ofn those who have the misfortune of getting COVID-19, which at this point in time, is almost the whole world.

The Pentagon's medical research arm, however, did credit the use of tobacco plants in 2012 for the quick development of 10 million doses of flu vaccine. Who knows whether tobacco will become a health improvement agent?

The official word is that there is no cure for the Coronavirus COVID-19. If there were a cure, the pandemic would be over already. But, the fact is there is no cure. If hydroxychloroquine is a cure, it is not recognized by the US health officials as such and so that's all we've got so far. In later chapters we show the therapeutics and types of "cures" from the Mayo Clinic. It is surely worth a scan.

We spent the first chapters discussing the cause of the pandemic and now it is time to discuss what we can do about it, even though there is no official cure.

The work has been going on and companies kept getting closer and closer and finally they developed three vaccines in record time and the FDA gave the vaccines emergency use authorizations. EUA.

A fairly comprehensive list of drugs for COVID-19 is presented at the following URL:

https://www.clinicaltrialsarena.com/analysis/coronavirus-mers-cov-drugs/

This chapter is based mostly on this work. As a non-scientist, the list of potential cures for this virus is amazingly large. Reading the blurbs gives one an idea of the complexity of the mission and the innovative approaches that are being developed to attack this killer virus.

You will see that there are a lot of facts on the cures already in the pipeline and there are more introduced every day. There are so many potential cures that if they all worked well, it would still be difficult to pick one. The fact is that there is hope that before mankind is eradicated by any strange disease, the geniuses out there will have a cure for us all.

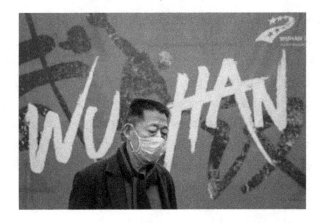

Despite no official cures, there are a number of wannabe cures. Like all things, some are good, some are bad, but other than the developer of a particular cure, none are fully advocated by the independent experts in the scientific community such as Dr. Fauci.

Now that Dr. Fauci's credibility has been diminished from leaning too far to the Democrat political side and being too cozy with China and WHO, and there being some public evidence that his lab may have contributed to the *gain of function* program that caused the disease in the first place, Fauci's standing in regular American circles is no longer the best.

Nonetheless, it helps one's spirit to know that scientists are already working on cures for Coronavirus and many believe there cures are ready for evaluation. That evaluation of course is what may take much more time than the brainwork to develop a cure.

After the SARS and MERS outbreaks, the National Institute of Health (NIH) immediately got to work funding potential cures. Even this long after the virus first struck, none of the cures are deemed ready for prime time yet. However, when there is a deep need like now, it adds impetus to efforts that may have been lagging for some time. The scientists get inspired to make something click after getting the proverbial shot in the arm such as a new pressing need.

The potential cures come from companies and organizations from all over the world, even from the country where the virus was first discovered. For example, the first COVID-19 vaccine in China is was ready for clinical trials by the end of April 2020, according to Xu Nanping, China's vice-minister of science and technology. Experts say a vaccine needs at least five years to mature enough to be released as safe and proven. Nonetheless, it all starts with a thesis that must be proven or disproven. Inovio Pharmaceuticals plans to begin clinical trials on their coronavirus vaccine this month—yes of this year—April this year.

Moderna, Pfizer, and J&J beat the odds but even they do not have full approval yet from the FDA.

Back in mid-2020, regular people on the street would not have been surprised if a vaccine were available shortly but those familiar with the process think that the most optimistic estimate of 18-months is even way too ambitious. That makes the availability of the vaccine before the end of 2020 and even more monumental achievement. So, though we have all these named therapeutic cures, there is nobody who has come forth to announce that any are the beat-all and end all.

Health officials from W.H.O. have noted that Gilead's remdesivir has demonstrated efficacy in treating the coronavirus infection. That does not make it the game changer or the scientific community would be touting it as such. First of all it can only be administered in a hospital.

Chloroquine approved for emergency use by US FDA

For a year or so now, ever since I heard the low-down on the French study and the success of the patients in the study, my favorite above all the unproven drugs has been Chloroquine and its derivative Hydroxychloroquine. President Trump tuned into the same study that I reference here and he asked the FDA to look into it as a therapeutic remedy to stop COVID-19 in its tracks after it has infected somebody.

Of course politically speaking the Never-Trumpers had a field-day bad mouthing the potential for a game changer because they feared the President might gain some electability credits from it.

For President Trump, whether Covid-19 patients should take a once-obscure malaria drug is not even a close call: "What do you have to lose?" he said during a briefing over a year ago "And a lot of people are saying that, and are taking it." I know I would if I caught the disease. I am fully double vaccinated but who knows with the variants.

For physicians on the frontlines, the question of whether to use that drug or other unproven medicines is among the most challenging they've faced: They're trained to make decisions based on rigorous data but have little to go on in treating patients with an entirely new disease. The claim that the results of studies in which none of the patients were denied the drug are not scientific and though in referenced published studies, the patients did well, because the clinical scientific method was not used, they declare the results anecdotal, meaning invalid for scientific purposes.

Based on Trump's urging, however, and despite Dr. Fauci's concern for the science of testing, The US Food and Drug Administration (FDA) looked at these two drugs and approved limited emergency use for chloroquine and hydroxychloroquine as a treatment for COVID-19. Later more than likely with pressure from Fauci and others the FDA pulled back its temporary OK of the drug.

FDA cautions against use of hydroxychloroquine or chloroquine for COVID-19 outside of the hospital setting or a clinical trial due to risk of heart rhythm problems

The FDA announced that this does not affect FDA-approved uses for malaria, lupus, and rheumatoid arthritis.

I don't know about you but this sounds fishy. No doctor of whom I am aware in my circles and those I follow have stopped prescribing hydroxychloroquine or Plaquenil (brand name for hydroxychloroquine) for Lupus because of the "risk for heart rhythm problems." If COVID is a killer and it is, why would you not want something that does not kill malaria patients or Lupus patients. If it does not kill them, chances are it won't kill COVID patients either and it just may help as thousands of doctors have determined.

Of course to have a doctor prescribe it, it may have to be under a diagnosis of malaria to get some pharmacies to fill it. Yes, folks, that is how political it has become. Trump likes hydroxychloroquine therefore it is bad. Humph!

The President of the United States, Donald Trump, had announced on 19 March that chloroquine and hydroxychloroquine, also known as Plaquenil, used to treat malaria, arthritis, and Lupus were approved by the FDA to be tested as a treatment for COVID-19. I don't recall seeing them formally stop the treatment but it seems that they have. Ask your doctor.

Chloroquine has endured many clinical trials conducted by government agencies and academic institutions and New York hospitals. Hydroxychloroquine is a derivative. It is my favorite of all the hopefuls because it has those anecdotal studies as backup, and doctors swearing it has helped their patients. President Trump was so confident that he had acquired over 300 million doses for the US stockpile as soon as he heard that it might be in short supply as it was about to become a preferred treatment outside the US.

Is this evidence from Dr. Smith non-anecdotal? You decide. He has already decided.

Laura Ingraham has a section on her show that she calls her Medicine Cabinet. It discusses the effectiveness of hydroxychloroquine, whether diabetes increases COVID-19 risk.

Drs. Ramin Oskoui, cardiologist and CEO of Foxhall cardiology, and Stephen Smith, founder of the Smith Center for Infectious Diseases and Urban Health, join Laura Ingraham on 'The Ingraham Angle.' almost every night to offer their perspectives and review new facts.

Dr. Stephen Smith, founder of The Smith Center for Infectious Diseases and Urban Health, said on "The Ingraham Angle" in early April 2020 that he is optimistic about the use of antimalarial medications and antibiotics to treat COVID-19 patients, calling it "a game-changer." Nobody put words in the Doctor's mouth. Nobody has disproven his theory

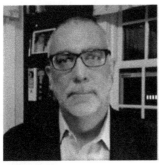 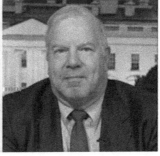

Dr. Smith   Dr. Oskoui

Ingraham's 'Medicine Cabinet' on effectiveness of hydroxychloroquine, whether diabetes increase COVID-19 risk

Dr. Smith was so encouraged and the results on his patients that he pronounced over a year ago:

"I think this is the beginning of the end of the pandemic. I'm very serious," Smith, an infectious disease specialist, told host of the Fox show, Laura Ingraham.

Currently there is no known cure for the coronavirus pandemic ravaging the globe.

Smith, who was treating 72 COVID-19 patients at the time he was interviewed said that he has been treating "everybody with hydroxychloroquine and azithromycin [an antibiotic]. We've been doing so for a while."

Dr. Smith pointed out that not a single COVID-19 patient of his that has been on the hydroxychloroquine and azithromycin regimen for five days or more has had to be intubated (go on a ventilator).

"The chance of that occurring by chance, according to my sons Leon and Hunter who did some stats for me, are .000-something," he said, adding that "it's ridiculously low."

Smith explained that "intubation means actually putting a tube down into your trachea and then you're placed on the ventilator for respiratory support."

As noted in 2020 when Dr. Smith made his statement, The Food and Drug Administration had recently announced an emergency-use authorization for several drugs, including hydroxychloroquine and chloroquine, despite a lack of clear scientific clinical trial-type evidence of their effectiveness. The drug has been used for malaria for 65 years with minimal issues.

A study published earlier this month by French researchers suggested that COVID-19 patients could be treated with antimalarial medication and antibiotics in the battle against the novel coronavirus.

Smith noted on Wednesday that he thinks his data supports the French study.

"Now you actually have an intra-cohort comparison saying that this regimen works," he told the show's host.

Speaking on "Fox & Friends" the same week as Dr. Smith, Dr. Mehmet Oz brought up an "important randomized study still unpublished from Wuhan, China."

He said that his team spoke to the medical leadership in China and vetted the study.

"We think it's real," Dr. Oz said on Thursday.

He then went on to explain what the study, which looked at 62 patients, showed. He noted that half of the patients got the traditional therapy being offered in China and the other half got the traditional therapy plus hydroxychloroquine. Technically, though the sample of 62 is small, it is not insignificant and it can be thought of as a valid clinical trial.

"In terms of symptoms, their temperatures, their fevers broke instead of three days, which is the norm over there on this treatment, they got two days," Dr. Oz said.

He added that "in terms of coughing, the other big symptom you have, again it takes a little over three days oftentimes for that to go away and that was dropped at two days."

Dr. Oz then pointed out the part that "really caught my attention."

"They did CT scans of the chest in all the patients. All the patients had pneumonia when they started. Over the course of the five-day treatment with the hydroxychloroquine and 55 percent of the control population where they just got the normal therapy there was resolve and resolution of the pneumonia in 81 percent of the patients on the hydroxychloroquine, there was improvement in the lung's images," he pointed out.

Dr. Oz noted that these results are "statistically significant." Clearly among the experts and among those second-guessing the experts, there has been a lot of guessing.

He went on to say that even though the study only monitored a small group of people, "they still got the measures that we like to see."

Dr. Oz acknowledged that a bigger clinical trial is still needed, adding that the Chinese study "is an early effort to try to show a lot of people whether this is the right way or the wrong way to go."

"I should point out in the 31 patients that were the control group, four patients had bad outcomes, they got significantly worse. None of the patients in the hydroxychloroquine group got significantly worse," he said.

"So the Chinese are using this as part of their routine treatment. They have a national protocol for measuring COVID-19. I think we ought to consider something like that in this country, but at least physicians and patients should be able to discuss this a bit more comfortably until we have the bigger randomized data from studies done in this country."

Other potential COVID-19 "cures" are being introduced

Other antiviral drugs are also planned to be fast-tracked for testing for coronavirus. There is a major impetus for those with a means to direct their resources into finding a solution to this plague on America. Not all the work is being gone in the US. For example Favilavir is the first approved coronavirus drug in China.

Favilavir

The National Medical Products Administration of China has approved the use of Favilavir, an anti-viral drug, as a treatment for coronavirus. The drug has reportedly shown efficacy in treating the disease with minimal side effects in a clinical trial involving 70 patients. The clinical trial was conducted in Shenzhen, Guangdong province.

There are many pharmaceutical companies involved in developing coronavirus drugs / vaccines. This gives us all hope yet, none have been mainstreamed as being the "cure." So we must all wait for all of the approvals to come in.

Here is a list of about thirty novel coronavirus drugs that pharmaceutical companies across the world are working on. The first grouping I show are candidate vaccines and are not therapeutic drugs such as hydroxychloroquine. I have included a short abstract from the web site above that describes the drug and how it is to work. Since I am not a doctor, I can say that they all have the potential to become major coronavirus vaccines or antivirals, etc. for treating the contagious coronavirus infection.

Novel coronavirus vaccines

Listed below are some of the coronavirus vaccines etc. in various stages of development, across the world.

Fusogenix DNA vaccine by Entos Pharmaceuticals

Entos Pharmaceuticals is in the process of developing what they call Fusogenix DNA vaccine developed using the Fusogenix drug delivery platform. It is designed to prevent COVID-19 infections. Fusogenix drug delivery platform is a proteo-lipid vehicle that introduces a genetic payload of "cure" directly into the cells.

Entos is working on developing an optimized payload containing multiple protein epitopes derived from SARS-COV-2 proteins. The objective is for these to stimulate an immune response in the body to prevent COVID-19 infection.

ChAdOx1 nCoV-19 by University of Oxford

The University of Oxford's ChAdOx1 nCoV-19 is an adenovirus vaccine vector developed by the university's Jenner Institute. The university is testing the vaccine in a clinical trial planned to be conducted in the Thames Valley Region.

Approximately 510 volunteers aged between 18 years and 55 years will be enrolled for the study.

Gimsilumab by Roivant Sciences

Roivant Sciences is advancing the development of Gimsilumab a clinical-stage, human monoclonal antibody. The drug targets granulocyte-macrophage colony stimulating factor (GM-CSF), which is a pro-inflammatory cytokine found in high levels in the serum of COVID-19 patients.

Targeting GM-CSF is expected to reduce lung damage and reduce mortality rate in COVID-19 patients.

AdCOVID by Altimmune

Altimmune has collaborated with the University of Alabama at Birmingham (UAB) to develop a single dose intranasal vaccine for COVID-19 named AdCOVID. The company is currently carrying out immunogenicity studies after, which phase one clinical trial material will be developed.

Altimmune and UAB will work with researchers to conduct preclinical animal studies and phase one clinical trial in the third quarter of 2020.

TJM2 by I-Mab Biopharma

I-Mab Biopharma by TJM2 It is a neutralizing antibody, as a treatment for cytokine storm in patients suffering from a severe case of coronavirus infection. The drug targets the human granulocyte-macrophage colony-stimulating factor (GM-CSF), which is responsible for acute and chronic inflammation.

The company will commence development after receiving approval for the Investigational New Drug (IND) application from the U.S. Food and Drug Administration (FDA).

Coronavirus vaccine by Medicago

Medicago is developing drug candidates against COVID-19 after having produced Virus-Like Particles (VLP) of the coronavirus. The company has formed a collaboration with Laval University's Infectious Disease Research Centre to develop antibodies against SARS-CoV-2.

The company's research activities are being partly funded by the Canadian Institutes for Health Research (CIHR).

AT-100 by Airway Therapeutics

Airway Therapeutics is exploring its novel human recombinant protein named AT-100 (rhSP-D) as a treatment for coronavirus. The company has announced a filing with the Respiratory Diseases Branch of the National Institutes of Health to evaluate the drug.

AT-100 has shown efficacy in preclinical studies in reducing inflammation and infection in the lungs, while also generating an immune response against various respiratory diseases.

TZLS-501 by Tiziana Life Sciences

Tiziana Life Sciences is developing its monoclonal antibody named TZLS-501 for the treatment of COVID-19. TZLS-501 is a human anti-interleukin-6 receptor (IL-6R), which helps in preventing lung damage and elevated levels of IL-6.

The drug works by binding to IL-6R and depleting the amount of IL-6 circulating in the body thereby reducing chronic lung inflammation.

OYA1 by OyaGen

OyaGen's OYA1 has shown strong antiviral efficacy against coronavirus in laboratory essays. It was found to be more effective than chlorpromazine HCl in inhibiting SARS-CoV-2 from replicating in cell culture.

OYA1 was earlier approved as an investigational new drug for treating cancer but abandoned due to lack of efficacy. OyaGen plans to conduct further research on the drug to determine the efficacy in treating coronavirus.

BPI-002 by BeyondSpring

BeyondSpring's BPI-002 is a small molecule agent indicated for treating various infections including COVID-19. It has the ability to activate CD4+ helper T cells and CD8+ cytotoxic T cells and generating an immune response in the body.

If combined with another COVID-19 vaccine, the drug has the ability to generate long-term protection against viral infections. BeyondSpring has filed US patent protection for the drug for treating viral infections.

Altimmune's intranasal coronavirus vaccine

An intranasal Covid-19 vaccine is being developed by US-based clinical-stage biopharmaceutical company, Altimmune.

Design and synthesis of the single-dose vaccine have been completed, while animal testing will follow.

The coronavirus vaccine is being developed based on a vaccine technology platform that is similar to NasoVAX, an influenza vaccine developed by Altimmune.

INO-4800 by Inovio Pharmaceuticals and Beijing Advaccine Biotechnology

Inovio Pharmaceuticals has collaborated with Beijing Advaccine Biotechnology Company to advance the development of the former's vaccine, INO-4800, as a novel coronavirus vaccine. The company has started pre-clinical testing for clinical product manufacturing.

The vaccine development is supported by a $9m grant from the Coalition for Epidemic Preparedness Innovations (CEPI).

Inovio announced an accelerated timeline for the development of the vaccine on 03 March. Preclinical trials are ongoing and the design for human clinical trials have been completed. The company has also prepared 3,000 doses for human clinical trials planned to be conducted across the US, China, and South Korea. Plans for large-scale manufacturing have also been developed.

Human clinical trials in 30 healthy volunteers are expected to commence in April 2020 in the US, followed by China, and South Korea. A phase one clinical trial is planned to be conducted in parallel in China, by Beijing Advaccine. Results from the clinical trials are expected to be available in September 2020.

Inovio aims to produce one million doses of the vaccine by the end of 2020 to perform additional clinical trials or emergency use.

NP-120 (Ifenprodil) by Algernon Pharmaceuticals

Algernon Pharmaceuticals has announced that it is exploring its NP-120 (Ifenprodil) as a potential treatment COVID-19. Ifenprodil is an N-methyl-d-aspartate (NDMA) receptor glutamate receptor antagonist sold under the brand name Cerocal. It has demonstrated efficacy in improving survivability in mice infected with H5N1.

APN01 by University of British Columbia and APEIRON Biologics

A drug candidate developed by APEIRON Biologics named APN01 is being tested in China in a phase one pilot trial as a treatment for COVID-19. APN01 is based on research conducted by a professor at the University of British Columbia for treating SARS. The research revealed that the ACE2 protein was the main receptor for the SARS virus.

The clinical trial will test the drug's efficacy in reducing the viral load in patients. Data from the trial will be used to determine if additional clinical trials are required to be conducted in larger number of patients.

mRNA-1273 vaccine by Moderna and Vaccine Research Center

Moderna and the Vaccine Research Center, a unit of the National Institute of Allergy and Infectious Diseases (NIAID), have collaborated to develop a vaccine for coronavirus. The vaccine targets the Spike (S) protein of the coronavirus.

The first vials of the vaccine have been manufactured at Moderna's Massachusetts manufacturing plant and shipped to NIAID for phase one human clinical trial. The trial began on 16 March at the Kaiser Permanente Washington Health Research Institute in Seattle, Washington. A total of 45 males and females aged between 18 and 45 have been enrolled for the trial.

The participants will be divided into three cohorts who will be administered 25 microgram (mcg), 100mcg or 250mcg dose 28 days apart.

Avian Coronavirus Infectious Bronchitis Virus (IBV) vaccine by MIGAL Research Institute

The MIGAL Research Institute in Israel announced that an Infectious Bronchitis Virus (IBV) vaccine developed to treat avian coronavirus has been modified to treat COVID-19. The vaccine has demonstrated efficacy in pre-clinical trials conducted by the Volcani Institute.

The IBV vaccine was developed after four years of research and has high genetic similarity to the human coronavirus. The institute has genetically modified the vaccine to treat COVID-19 and will be available in the oral form.

The institute is currently exploring potential partners for producing the vaccine in the next eight to ten weeks and obtaining the necessary safety approvals for in-vivo testing.

TNX-1800 by Tonix Pharmaceuticals

Tonix Pharmaceuticals has partnered with Southern Research, a non-profit research organization, to develop a vaccine for coronavirus named TNX-1800. The vaccine is a modified horsepox virus developed using Tonix's proprietary horsepox vaccine platform.

TNX-1800 is designed to express a protein derived from the virus that causes the coronavirus infection. Southern Research will be responsible for evaluating the efficacy of the vaccine, under the partnership.

Brilacidin by Innovation Pharmaceuticals

Innovation Pharmaceuticals announced that it is evaluating Brilacidin, a defensin mimetic drug candidate, as a potential treatment for coronavirus. Brilacidin has shown antibacterial, anti-inflammatory and immunomodulatory properties in several clinical trials.

The company is planning to explore research collaborations and seek federal grants to develop the coronavirus drug. It is already investigating the drug for inflammatory bowel disease and oral mucositis in cancer patients.

Innovation has signed two material transfer agreements with a university in the US and 12 biocontainment labs in the US for evaluation of Brilacidin as a treatment for COVID-19. One of the biocontainment labs is scheduled to commence testing of the drug in the third week of March.

Recombinant subunit vaccine by Clover Biopharmaceuticals

Clover Biopharmaceuticals is developing a recombinant subunit vaccine using its patented Trimer-Tag© technology. The company is developing the vaccine based on the trimeric S protein (S-Trimer) of the COVID-19 coronavirus, which is responsible for binding with the host cell and causing a viral infection.

Using Trimer-Tag© technology, Clover successfully produced the subunit vaccine in a mammalian cell-culture based expression system on 10 February. The company also identified antigen-specific antibody in the serum of fully recovered patients who were previously infected by the virus.

A highly purified form of the S-Trimer vaccine is expected to be available in six to eight weeks for performing pre-clinical studies. The company is equipped with in-house cGMP biomanufacturing capabilities to scale-up production if the vaccine is proven to be successful.

Clover is also collaborating with GSK to develop a vaccine using the latter's pandemic adjuvant system.

Vaxart's coronavirus vaccine

Vaxart is developing an oral recombinant vaccine in tablet formulation using its proprietary oral vaccine platform, VAAST.

The company plans to develop vaccines based on the published genome of 2019-nCOV to be tested in pre-clinical models for mucosal and systemic immune responses.

CytoDyn-leronlimab's (PRO-140)

CytoDyn is examining leronlimab (PRO 140), a CCR5 antagonist, as a potential coronavirus drug.

The drug is already being investigated in phase two clinical trials as a treatment for HIV and has been awarded fast-track approval status by the United States Food and Drug Administration.

Linear DNA Vaccine by Applied DNA Sciences and Takis Biotech.

Applied DNA Sciences' subsidiary LineaRx and Takis Biotech formed a joint venture on 07 February to develop a linear DNA vaccine as a treatment for coronavirus. The JV will use Polymerase Chain Reaction (PCR)-based DNA manufacturing technology to develop the vaccine.

The PCR technology offers several advantages including high purity, increased production speed, and absence of antibiotics and bacterial contaminants. Further, the vaccine gene developed through this technology can be effective without being inserted into the patient's genome.

The design for four DNA vaccine candidates is expected to be produced using the PCR technology for carrying out animal testing. The design of one of the vaccine candidates is based on the entire spike gene of the coronavirus, while the remaining are designed based on the antigenic portions of the protein.

BXT-25 by BIOXYTRAN to treat late-stage acute respiratory distress syndrome (ARDS)

BIOXYTRAN announced that it is exploring partners to develop its lead drug candidate, BX-25, as a treatment for Acute Respiratory Distress Syndrome (ARDS) in late-stage patients infected with the coronavirus. The diffusion of oxygen to the blood is comprised in patients suffering from ARDS leading to fluid build-up in the lungs.

BX-25 is designed to be 5,000 times smaller than blood cells and efficiently transport oxygen through the body for a period of nine hours before being processed by the liver. The drug can help in supplying oxygen to the vital organs and enable the patient to recover and survive.

MERS CoV vaccines for coronavirus

Novavax's MERS coronavirus vaccine candidate

Novavax developed a novel Middle East Respiratory Syndrome (MERS) coronavirus vaccine candidate in 2013, post the identification of the first MERS coronavirus ((MERS-CoV) in Saudi Arabia in 2012. It is a crucial target for vaccine development by the Coalition for Epidemic Preparedness Innovations (CEPI) and is a priority disease for the World Health Organization (WHO).

The candidate is designed to primarily bind to the major surface S-protein and developed using the company's recombinant nanoparticle vaccine technology. Tested along with the Novavax's proprietary adjuvant Matrix-M™, it inhibited infection by inducing immune responses in the laboratory studies.

Novavax has received $4m in funding from CEPI to advance the development of the vaccine. The company has produced several nanoparticle vaccine candidates for testing in animal models and aims to carry out human trials in 2020.

The MERS coronavirus is related to the severe acute respiratory syndrome (SARS) coronavirus, for which the company had previously developed a recombinant nanoparticle vaccine candidate.

Inovio Pharma's INO-4700

The investigational DNA immunotherapy, INO-4700 (GLS-5300) is being developed by Inovio in partnership with GeneOne Life Science.

It is delivered as vaccine intramuscularly, using the Cellectra® delivery device.

The company has received a $5m grant from the Bill and Mellinda Gates foundation to accelerate the development of the Cellectra® delivery device.

The vaccine was well-tolerated and demonstrated high immune responses against the MERS-CoV in 94% of patients in the early-stage clinical trial in July 2019.

It also generated broad-based T cell responses in 88% of the subjects.

"Research organizations such as the National Institutes of Health (NIH), US are also developing a vaccine for the coronavirus."

Coronavirus drugs

The novel coronavirus drugs in various stages of development globally are listed below.

Remdesivir (GS-5734) by Gilead Sciences

An Ebola drug developed by Gilead Sciences that was found to be ineffective is now being tested in two phase III randomized clinical trials in Asian countries.

The trials are being performed on 761 patients in a randomized, placebo-controlled, double-blind study at multiple hospitals in Wuhan, the epicenter of the novel coronavirus outbreak. The results from the trials are expected to be available over the next few weeks.

According to a report by The New England Journal of Medicine (NEJM), remdesivir, when administered to a coronavirus patient in the US, appeared to have improved the clinical condition.

The University of Nebraska Medical Center is also carrying out clinical trials to test the safety and efficacy of the drug. The first patient to be administered the drug is an evacuee from the Diamond Princess cruise ship.

Actemra by Roche to treat coronavirus-related complications

China approved the use of Roche's Actemra for the treatment of severe complications related to coronavirus. Drugs like Actemra have the ability to prevent cytokine storms or overreaction of the immune system, which is considered as the main reason behind organ failure leading to death in some coronavirus patients.

Actemra is also being evaluated in a clinical trial in China, which is expected to enroll 188 coronavirus patients. The clinical trial is expected to be conducted until May 10.

Biocryst Pharma's Galidesivir,

This is a potential antiviral for coronavirus treatment

The antiviral drug Galidesivir (BCX4430) has shown broad-spectrum activity against a wide range of pathogens including coronavirus. It is a nucleoside RNA polymerase inhibitor that disrupts the process of viral replication.

The drug has already shown survival benefits in patients against deadly viruses such as Ebola, Zika, Marburg, and Yellow fever.

Galidesivir is currently in advanced development stage under the Animal Rule to combat multiple potential viral threats including coronaviruses, flaviviruses filoviruses, paramyxoviruses, togaviruses, bunyaviruses, and arenaviruses.

Regeneron's REGN3048-3051 and Kevzara

Discovered by Regeneron, the combination of neutralizing monoclonal antibodies REGN3048 and REGN3051 is being studied against coronavirus infection in a first-in-human clinical trial sponsored by the National Institute of Allergy and Infectious Diseases (NIAID). The safety and tolerability of the drug will be studied in 48 patients.

Both the antibodies bind to S-protein of MERS coronavirus. The intravenous administration of the drug in the mouse model of MERS resulted in the high-level neutralization of the MERS coronavirus in circulating blood with reduced viral loads in the lungs.

Regeneron has partnered with Sanofi to evaluated Kevzara, a fully-human monoclonal antibody, in a phase two/three clinical trial in patients with severe COVID-19 infection. Kevzara is approved for the treatment of rheumatoid arthritis and is known to block the interleukin-6 (IL-6) pathway, which causes an overactive inflammatory response in the lungs of COVID-19 patients.

SNG001 by Synairgen Research

Synairgen Research's SNG001, an inhaled drug, is planned to be tested by the University of Southampton to treat asthma, chronic obstructive pulmonary disease and lower respiratory tract illnesses caused by coronavirus.

SNG001 is a formulation of naturally occurring Interferon-β, which is administered through a nebulizer and is delivered directly to the lungs to reduce the severity of the infection caused by coronavirus.

AmnioBoost by Lattice Biologics

Lattice Biologics is exploring the efficacy of its amniotic fluid concentrate, AmnioBoost, in treating acute respiratory distress syndrome (ARDS) in COVID-19 patients. AmnioBoost was developed for chronic adult inflammatory conditions such as osteoarthritis.

The drug has shown efficacy in reducing the inflammatory conditions caused by several diseases including coronavirus. It reduces the production of pro-inflammatory cytokines while boosting the production of anti-inflammatory cytokines.

Other companies developing coronavirus vaccines/drugs
Inovio Pharmaceuticals, Moderna, and Novavax
Companies such as Inovio Pharmaceuticals, Moderna, and Novavax

have been reported to be developing vaccines. A total of 30 therapies are being tested, including few traditional medicines for coronavirus treatment by Chinese scientists. Chloroquine phosphate has shown efficacy in treating symptoms of the disease, among the 30 therapies. Patients administered with the drug achieved a better drop in fever and shorter recovery time in clinical trials being conducted in hospitals in the Guangdong province and Hunan province.

Enanta Pharmaceuticals

Enanta Pharmaceuticals has announced its plans to develop antiviral drug candidates to treat COVID-19 patients. The company is testing compounds from its existing antiviral compound library for potential efficacy in treating COVID-19. It has also launched a drug discovery program to develop direct-acting drug candidates to treat COVID-19.

Predictive Oncology

Predictive Oncology has launched an AI Platform for the discovery and development of vaccines against coronavirus. The company has signed an agreement with InventaBioTech to acquire Soluble Therapeutics, which provides it with access to the HSCTM Technology.

Predictive will use the HSCTM Technology along with its predictive modeling platform to deploy an AI discovery platform that can screen the ideal combination of additives and excipients for protein formulations.

Emergent BioSolutions

Emergent BioSolutions is developing two plasma-derived product candidates or hyperimmunes using its hyperimmune platforms for the treatment of coronavirus. The hyperimmune platforms have been used previously for the development of several approved products including vaccines for smallpox, botulism, and anthrax.

The hyperimmunes are polyclonal antibodies derived from plasma, which are capable of generating an immune response and protecting against infection. Product candidate derived from human plasma is named COVID-HIG, while COVID-EIG is derived from equine plasma. Both will be explored for the treatment of patients with a severe case of infection.

Integral Molecular

Integral Molecular has launched a vaccine program using its two technology platforms including Shotgun Mutagenesis Epitope Mapping and the Membrane Proteome Array. The technologies will help in understanding the human immune response to the coronavirus and isolate the cellular receptors that enable the virus to spread quickly.

The Shotgun technology helps in identifying more than 1,000 binding sites for antibodies, while the Membrane Proteome Array technology is capable of identifying the receptors through which viruses infect cells.

CEL-SCI

CEL-SCI is developing immunotherapy against COVID-19 using its proprietary LEAPS peptide technology, which utilizes conserved areas of the coronavirus proteins to generate T-cell responses and reduce viral load. The technology can also be used to develop immunotherapeutic peptides with both antiviral and anti-inflammatory properties.

The peptides developed using this technology can help in reducing tissue damage from inflammation caused due to lung infection, which is a major cause of mortality in elderly patients.

AJ Vaccines

AJ Vaccines has launched the development of a vaccine against COVID-19. The company will use the latest technology to develop antigens that can mimic the native structures of the virus. The vaccine will be capable of inducing a strong immune response in the body thereby protecting against the infection.

Takeda Pharmaceutical Company

Takeda Pharmaceutical Company has announced plans to develop a plasma-derived therapy against coronavirus. The anti-SARS-CoV-2 polyclonal hyperimmune globulin (H-IG) therapy will be designed to treat high-risk patients. The H-IG therapy includes concentrated pathogen-specific antibodies derived from plasma of recovered patients. These antibodies have the potential to generate an immune response when injected into a new patient.

Heat Biologics

Heat Biologics has announced plans to develop a vaccine to treat or prevent coronavirus infection using its proprietary gp96 vaccine platform. The technology is capable of reprogramming live cells to produce antigens that can bind to the gp96 protein and generate an immune response against those antigens.

Pfizer

Pfizer announced that it has identified certain under development antiviral compounds that may be effective in treating coronavirus. The company is planning to partner with a third party to screen and identify potential compounds by the end of March and begin testing in April.

Mateon Therapeutics

Mateon Therapeutics has launched an antiviral response program to develop coronavirus treatments using its therapeutic and artificial intelligence (AI) platforms. It has also established a division, which will adopt a multi-modal approach to developing COVID-19 treatments as well as other future zootonic outbreaks.

Hong Kong University of Science and Technology

The Hong Kong University of Science and Technology has identified several vaccine targets, which can be developed as a treatment for coronavirus. Researchers at the university have identified B-cell and T-cell epitopes, which are capable of generating an immune response against the SARS virus and a similar response against the coronavirus.

Some of the epitopes identified may be capable of generating an immune response specifically against COVID-19.

Generex

Generex has announced that it is developing a COVID-19 vaccine following a contract from a Chinese consortium comprising of China Technology Exchange, Beijing Zhonghua Investment Fund Management, Biology Institute of Shandong Academy of Sciences and Sinotek-Advocates International Industry Development.

The company will utilize its Ii-Key immune system activation technology to produce a COVID-19 peptide for human clinical trials.

Generex will receive an upfront payment of $1m to commence the groundwork for the vaccine development and $5m licensing fee for its Ii-Key technology. It is also eligible to receive a 20% royalty on every dose of vaccine produced under the contract.

Columbia University

Researchers at Columbia University have been awarded a $2.1m grant by the Jack Ma Foundation to develop a cure for coronavirus. Four different teams at the university will adopt various approaches towards the development of a vaccine against coronavirus.

Vaccine by Tulane University

Tulane University has launched a research program to identify a potential coronavirus medicine in the form of a vaccine. The university will utilize a grant from the Brown Foundation to carry out the research activities.

ImmunoPrecise Antibodies

ImmunoPrecise Antibodies has launched a vaccine and therapeutic antibody program to develop a vaccine as well as antibodies against COVID-19. The company will use its B Cell Select™ and DeepDisplay™ discovery platforms to therapeutic compounds against the coronavirus.

The company has updated its research efforts and noted that it will be using the PolyTope mAb TherapyTM and EVQLV's artificial intelligence platforms develop a COVID-19 therapy.

Serum Institute of India

Serum Institute of India (SII) is collaborating with Codagenix, a US-based biopharmaceutical company, to develop a cure for coronavirus using a vaccine strain similar to the original virus. The vaccine is currently in the pre-clinical testing phase, while human trials are expected to commence in the next six months. SII is expected to launch the vaccine in the market by early 2022.

Southwest Research Institute

Southwest Research Institute is using its virtual screening called Rhodium to identify potential drug candidates for treating coronavirus from more than two million drug compounds. The most promising compounds will be identified for further development.

Zydus Cadila

Zydus Cadila announced the launch of an accelerated research program to develop a vaccine for COVID-19 using two novel approaches. The first approach includes the development of a DNA vaccine against the viral membrane protein of the virus, while a live attenuated recombinant measles virus (rMV) vectored vaccine will be developed in the second approach. The rMV-based vaccine works by inducing specific neutralizing antibodies, which will provide protection from the coronavirus infection.

NanoViricides

NanoViricides, a clinical-stage company, is working on developing a treatment for nCoV-2019 using its nanoviricide® technology. The company's technology is used to develop ligands that can bind to the virus in the same way as a cognate receptor and attack various points of the virus.

Vir Biotechnology

Vir Biotechnology, a clinical-stage immunology company, announced on 12 February that it has identified two monoclonal antibodies that can bind to the virus that causes COVID-19. The antibodies target the spike (S) protein of the virus by entering through the cellular receptor ACE2.

The company has formed a partnership with WuXi Biologics on 25 February to commercialize the antibodies identified to treat coronavirus. If approved, Wuxi will have the rights to market the therapies in China, while Vir will retain the marketing rights in other countries.

Vir has also partnered with Alnylam Pharmaceuticals to identify siRNA candidates targeting SARS-CoV-2. It has formed another partnership with Biogen for cell line and process development and manufacturing of the antibodies.

HIV drugs for coronavirus treatment

Abbvie's HIV protease inhibitor, lopinavir

is being studied along with ritonavir for the treatment of MERS and SARS coronaviruses. The repurposed drug is already approved for the treatment of HIV infection under the trade name Kaletra®.

The combination is listed in the WHO list of essential medicines. Lopinavir is believed to act on the intracellular processes of coronavirus replication and demonstrated reduced mortality in the non-human primates (NHP) model of the MERS.

Lopinavir/ritonavir in combination with ribavirin showed reduced fatality rate and milder disease course during an open clinical trial in patients in the 2003 SARS outbreak.

Cipla is also reportedly planning to repurpose its HIV drug LOPIMUNE, which is a combination of protease inhibitors Lopinavir and Ritonavir, for the treatment of coronavirus.

A licensed generic of Kaletra®, LOPIMUNE is currently available in packs of 60 tablets each, containing 200mg of Lopinavir and 50mg of Ritonavir.

Janssen Pharmaceutical Companies, a subsidiary of Johnson & Johnson, donated its PREZCOBIX® HIV medication (darunavir/cobicistat) for use in research activities aimed at finding a treatment for COVID-19.

Darunavir is a protease inhibitor marketed by Janssen. Anecdotal reports suggest darunavir as potentially having antiviral activity against COVID-19. It is, however, currently approved only for use with a boosting agent, and in combination with other antiretrovirals, for the treatment of HIV-1.

Janssen does not have in vitro or clinical data to support the use of darunavir as a treatment for COVID-19. The drug is in the process of being evaluated in vitro for any potential activity against the coronavirus.

Further, Janssen has partnered with the Biomedical Advanced Research and Development Authority (BARDA) to expedite the development of a COVID-19 treatment.

What will it take to beat the coronavirus?

Andy J. Semotiuk; Contributor. I write about investor immigration and about Immigration issues.

The battle with Covid-19 will require help from all of us What is the best way to deal with it?. Let's talk about the best way to deal with it—with or without a vaccine or therapeutic?

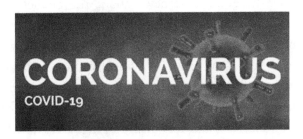

Coronavirus is a tough enemy to beat

The experts tell us that while the infections should peak in just a few weeks, the coronavirus pandemic could last for another 12 to 18 months. That's the bad news. The good news then was that it might have gone away in the summer. But it did not!

Regardless, at the time in 2020, as we know well, with all the companies racing to beat the competition for completing a vaccine, without a vaccine, we are all less safe. Some say that when we are free from the state's lockdown, the only real solution appears to be to develop a herd immunity.

What is herd immunity?

After at least half the population has had the infection, we ultimately become immune to it. In the Plague of 1918, the Spanish Flu, that took two or three years and nobody was sure if it would ever stop. There is no guarantee event that will work. Besides, without extensive testing, we have no idea what percentage of the population has been infected.

Alternatively, and hopefully most likely, a vaccine or a therapeutic will be developed and then widespread "inoculation" will take place. The experts tell us probably that could take a year or more if you are an optimist. Who knows?

Meanwhile, we have watched news about the challenges that the covid-19 virus has brought to America's health care system. Some of the revelations such as: American athletes getting tested while others wait in line, a 17-year old young man dying because a hospital would not treat him because of a lack of medical insurance, and America running out of ventilators and basic protective gear to treat patients for front line health care workers have been very discouraging. They have highlighted some of our worst moments. It seems like those type of incidents are already behind us.

Economically, the news that over twenty-two million applicants filed unemployment claims over the past four weeks and that the total unemployed in March of this year alone has risen to almost 20 million has been staggering. And that does not include the two or three million foreign workers who have likely become jobless suddenly as well-whether they are legal or illegal.

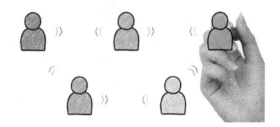

Social distancing is the recommendation that has saved us so far. When the herd immunity hits or Hydroxychloroquine is approved and works, we can let our guard down but not until. There is nothing else in the armament of medical science to beat this virus.

All these shocking developments have most Americans very concerned about whether. this will ever be over. Most are down so low, about 75% think it is going to go on for a long time to come even if it crashes the economy for good.

And Dr. Anthony Fauci, the government's top expert on infectious diseases, has cautioned that the virus dictates the timeline and warned that to gradually reopen the country we need to be able to execute widespread testing. The means to get this job done must be in place, so doctors can better identify, isolate and trace cases. He may be right but somebody has to hold the essential jobs and it is getting more difficult with the population being so skittish and with the hoarding mentality overriding the notion of herd immunization.

Despite all that, as America and the world address these seemingly insurmountable issues, there are a number of good things happening as well.

How We Are Adapting

For one thing, relationships between people are warmer, total strangers seem to be more polite, helpful and accommodating for the most part. Even when an outrageous act occurs, just a month or two ago, nobody would be alarmed. "It's how we are." However, just today, twenty cars had their tires slashed in a hospital ER parking lot. The deed was discovered when shift nurses tried to pull away after putting in a long shift. People on the scene in the hospitals and in the press rooms of the nation's media, treated this as one of the most egregious disgusting acts of the pandemic. They are right. People are beginning to care about people and such nasty treatment of care-givers is viewed as intolerable.

There is a better sense of community that has arisen as we care for one another. Perhaps it is just because we sense that there is the potential of mortal danger involved. There is the sense that we are equally vulnerable, although we are told that older people are more at risk.

Keeping a physical distance has required us to be more flexible in allowing others to go ahead of us, or pass us while we stand by. We are learning that we should wear non-medical face masks to protect one another from each other.

Isolated as we maybe, our televisions, radios, smart phones, and personal computers are helping us all learn new ways to interact with each another. For example, in my case I have been invited to participate a few Zoom calls. I am going to make sure that I can so next time I can say yes.

Before the outbreak, I never felt it worth my time to learn the technology and that meant I never used it. I will now. There is a dawning realization that we are more connected to each other than we realized previously. Globalization, in the sense that what the Chinese are doing affects what we are doing, as an example, is increasingly apparent to us.

There is other good news, if not just good points. Most people with COVID-19 recover. They get better. Estimates now suggest that in the neighborhood of 99% of people infected with COVID-19 will recover to lead normal lives. Children are infected less often and have milder symptoms. The CDC tells us all that vast majority of infections so far have afflicted adults., especially senior citizen adults. The number of new cases has plateaued in many places across the world including the US states. China and the Republic of Korea have reported significantly declining epidemics.

Is it not a great thing that we have the Internet. We are not alone. Those who stubbornly exist without the Internet have a good reason to reconsider. The "Net" is helping us communicate a lot with each other and even to medical providers.

People in isolation or quarantine can ask for help, visit friends, see family and doctors virtually, and provide updates on their condition. Our response to future pandemics should also improve because this one has exposed shortcomings in healthcare systems throughout the world, including the US.

This provides an opportunity for all of us to improve them. Many people and organizations have stepped up to help. Some major health insurers have promised to cover care and testing related to COVID-19, and some celebrities and professional athletes and even business people have donated significant resources to help those taking a financial hit because of the pandemic.

It's time to thank God and all the Helpers

Let us not forget to be thankful to all those who work daily in the front lines to save us - the doctors, nurses, lab technicians, first responders, police officers, fire fighters and all the others. Let us also be thankful for the tremendous leadership we have seen across the country by those who care for us and seek to marshal the resources needed to win this battle. It is refreshing to see President Trump in a positive light, like a caring godfather for everybody in the country on both sides of the aisle. Thank you President Trump for your Fireside Chats. FDR would be proud of you.

Above all, let us not forget our families and neighbors who are helping us daily and who constantly remind us of our humanity.

Life will get better

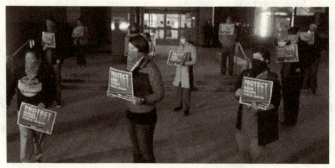

SAN FRANCISCO, CA - APRIL 2: UCSF nurses hold a rally before dawn to protest a lack of personal protection.
HEARST NEWSPAPERS VIA GETTY IMAGES

In short, we all have learned that this nasty pandemic has given us opportunities to re-imagine the world and our place in it. No doubt we will face even more challenges. But while we deal with the difficulties visited upon us and mourn our major losses, let us take note of the good that has entered our lives as well. You know that we will survive this challenge, no matter what it takes, and return to a different life hopefully better than the one we once had. Let's leave the bickering where it belongs—in the garbage.

CHAPTER 7

How to Resume Your Life

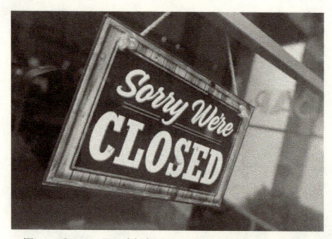

Times Square Establishment—A SIGN of the times

Should we stay closed and separated?

On April 10, four days before I wrote this chapter before I wrote some book revisions, the New York Times Magazine wrote a piece about restarting America. After a read of their article one would not necessarily conclude that we should ever restart when government is being so helpful to the people right now.

Here is how they began their article:

"The politics of the coronavirus have made it seem indecent to talk about the future. As President Trump has flirted with reopening America quickly— saying in late March that he'd like to see "packed churches" on Easter and returning to the theme days ago with "we cannot let this continue"— public-health experts have felt compelled to call out the dangers. Many Americans have responded by rejecting as monstrous the whole idea of any trade-off between saving lives and saving the economy. And in the near term, it's true that those two goals align: For the sake of both, it's imperative to keep businesses shuttered and people in their homes as much as possible.

In the longer run, though, it's important to acknowledge that a trade-off will emerge — and become more urgent in the coming months, as the economy slides deeper into recession. The staggering toll of unemployment has reached more than 22 million in just the last four weeks. There will be difficult compromises between doing everything possible to save lives from COVID-19 and preventing other life-threatening, or—altering, harms.

When can the US ethically bring people back to work and school and begin to resume the usual rhythms of American life? The times brought five people together in a video-conference and asked them point blank, what would it take to reopen America. Of course there is the current battle of who has the authority—the President or the fifty Governors. But, assuming that one will be solved, there is a lot of disagreement on when we should open. For eight governors, in fact, who have not issued stay-at home orders, the opening question is moot. They have not shut down.

If you want to see what the Times said about the subject, feel free to go to https://www.nytimes.com/2020/04/10/magazine/coronavirus-economy-debate.html. The panelists in their piece do not reflect my views on the subject. Bioethicist Ezekiel Emanuel adopted the "Whole

Lives" program for Obamacare. The "Death Panels" were part of his work in which if you were under ten or above fifty years old, Emanuel would serve you your health-care last.

He would not be on my panel. He is not pro-American in my opinion. His take is to keep America shut down until there is a vaccine, which he believes will be here in perhaps eighteen months. By then folks, if we stayed shut down with enhanced social distancing as in Michigan, China would own America. Therefore, I am not interested at all in the Emanuel Plan.

What if you knew that the number of deaths for the flu this year were more than four times the number of deaths from the coronavirus. It is by the way. In the U.S. alone, the flu this year (also called influenza) has caused an estimated 38 million illnesses, 390,000 hospitalizations and up to 62,000 deaths this season. Think about that. It's like that every year and we do not close down the country. At the time this was written, COVID-19 had caused about 29,000 deaths in the US this particular year because we hade no vaccine and would not accept the best therapeutic as our gold standard—hydroxychloroquine. Many experts say that the # of deaths would be significantly less if hydroxychloroquine were adopted as both a prophylaxis and as a possible cure.

Physicians use Hydroxychloroquine worldwide

Valerie Richardson of The Washington Times reported a week ago on Thursday, April 2, 2020 that an international poll of more than 6,000 doctors released Thursday found that the antimalarial drug hydroxychloroquine was the most highly rated treatment for the novel coronavirus. For me that means I want it if I am sick with the virus or as a prophylaxis.

The survey was conducted by Sermo, a global health care polling company, of 6,227 physicians in 30 countries. They found that 37%

of those treating COVID-19 patients rated hydroxychloroquine as the "most effective therapy" from a list of 15 options. These are doctors.

Of the physicians surveyed, 3,308 said they had either ordered a COVID-19 test or been involved in caring for a coronavirus patient, and 2,171 of those responded to the question asking which medications were most effective. Only when the scientific community accepts information such as this and offers real opinions about the positive aspects of its efficacy will this treatment get the full respect that it deserves from the world. Then, many real lives will be saved.

The activist press is against hydroxychloroquine after finding out that from the daily briefings that President Donald Trump authorized Peter Navarro to find thirty million or more doses from around the world from countries who had chosen not to export the medicine. Navarro found them and brought them to the stockpile. If Trump is for anything, the activist press is against it for no other reason.

President Donald Trump has expressed his interest in the merits of the anti-malarial drug hydroxychloroquine as a coronavirus game changing cure and as a prophylaxis. I learned about it from two doctors on the Laura Ingraham show and the evidence is compelling

Drs. Ramin Oskoui, cardiologist and CEO of Foxhall cardiology, and Stephen Smith, founder of the Smith Center for Infectious Diseases and Urban Health, told their story to Laura Ingraham on Fox News. The activist opposition press refute all of the evidence presented because they fear a cure for the coronavirus would assure a victory for Trump in the November elections. It is amazing that this activist opposition media does not care what happens to America as long as they can discredit the president.

Democrat Representative cured by hydroxychloroquine

Despite the opinion of the lying press, nonetheless, former coronavirus patients like actor Daniel Dae Kim and Michigan Democratic State Representative Karen Whitsett swear by it. However, even after receiving emergency FDA approval, the anti-malarial drug hydroxychloroquine still has an image problem on the political left after being touted by President Trump. When the left found Trump favored the drug, that was enough for them to be against it—unless of course they get the virus.

Democratic State Representative Karen Whitsett from Michigan has been telling anybody who will listen about her good news. She says that the controversial drug hydroxychloroquine stopped her coronavirus symptoms "within a couple hours."

The FDA issued the emergency-use authorization late on a particular Sunday early-on for chloroquine and its next-generation version, hydroxychloroquine, as treatments for the novel coronavirus, fueling the political back-and-forth that erupted March 19 when Mr. Trump called hydroxychloroquine a potential "game changer."

There is enough evidence for me that the drug is safe and effective as a cure and as a prophylaxis that I wrote two articles for my local paper. I was called the other day telling me that the first was about to be printed in the Citizens Voice.

With all of the fuss for the first month of the shutdown with hospitals and EMTs having mask shortages and doctors and nurses having to go to work without the proper PPE's (personal protective equipment, I penned this article

Here is the Short Letter in italics that I sent to the editor.

Date: Wed, 25 Mar 2020 19:11:59 -0400
From: "Brian W. Kelly"
Subject: What if we no longer needed N95 masks?

I have no medical credentials to be considered but I offer this anyway. My favorite poem by Emily Dickinson starts with I'm nobody, who are you? I know who I am.

In my whole career with IBM I was a problem solver. Problems that we did not know about yesterday, we had to solve today. When I get a problem in my head and possible solutions, I did not stop until my solution was proven wrong and I had to move on to possible solution #2, or 3, or whatever.

I am intrigued by the studied capabilities of hydroxychloroquine, an effective malaria drug to fight COVID-19. It is in clinical tests in NY since Tuesday but I hear nothing about it. In the French study that has been popularized by Dr. Oz, we know that the French have cured all members of their small study. It took one person a few days longer to show relaxed symptoms. But that person too was cured. Hydroxychloroquine is also seen as a great prophylaxis (preventative). It is used so that those heading to malaria infested countries do not contract malaria.

It is said anecdotally that it does the same for the coronavirus. In other words, it can prevent one from contracting the virus.

What if it works? Does anybody know? It seems like nobody at this point cares about its preventative abilities.

Think of it?

Until the major innovations in making N95 masks for hospital workers were developed, there was and there still may be a mask shortage.

What if hydroxychloroquine were such an effective prophylaxis for the virus that anybody who took the proper preventative dosage became immune from getting the virus?

What if?

How are problems solved but first with a thesis?

What if?

The N95 mask shortage would no longer matter if a simple pill or injection could prevent the virus from affecting hospital and other EMT workers.

Should we know more about this?

We could concentrate on respirators and testing!

--- End of letter ---

After a week, I added to the facts in the letter and sent it again

2nd letter to the editor about hydroxychloroquine

Date: Wed, 8 Apr 2020 07:11:34 -0400
From: "Brian W. Kelly"
Subject: Save lives with this new therapeutic remedy

Doctors themselves are taking chloroquine and hydroxychloroquine as a cure and as a prophylactic. The people should know about this.

Additionally, with the significant # of health care workers and EMS who have caught the virus in their work it would also help in keeping them safe.

Evidence that these drugs serve as an effective prophylactic is widespread. For 65 years, chloroquine has been used in Africa and various countries to fight malaria. Where the drug is used regularly, there are no cases of covid-19.

Additionally on a recent talk show two doctors discussed

Hydroxychloroquine, Azithromycin and zinc, in a dose they said costs about $20.00 can be used as a therapeutic cure for those moderately and even severely infected. The sooner one takes the medicine however, the better. Additionally, these doctors treat Lupus patients and Rheumatoid Arthritis Patients with the hydroxychloroquine and have been doing so for years without any patient going to the hospital because of the medicine.

The drug is safe. Additionally, the one doctor treats 2000 patients for Lupus and none have contracted COVID-19. He cited another study of 14,500 Lupus patients and none have COVID. This attests to its prophylaxis capabilities.

Locally on the Frank Andrews show yesterday, Louis called in to tell his story of contracting covid-19. He said he thought he would have no issue because he was young and strong and in good health but after ten days, he had not improved and began having breathing difficulties. After a few days he called 911 and was admitted to treat the coronavirus covid-19.

He was given breathing assistance with a ventilator and he thought he might not make it. Then, he was given

Hydroxychloroquine, zinc, and Azithromycin. After a day or so, he was taken off breathing assist and put on oxygen, then a reduced oxygen flow and after a few days he was discharged free of the virus. On death's door to on the way home. That is not anecdotal if you are Louis, that is very real.

A state Democrat representative from Michigan said she heard Donald Trump talking about the possibilities of the drug on TV in one of the updates. She had the virus and was getting worse. She asked her doctor if she could be put on the drug and he did so. In four hours, she told the audience she had no symptoms. Her Doctor was on the air with her.

I am thinking about when the US goes back to work. All of the serology testing for antibodies to see who is immune we know will take forever. America recently brought in 329,000,000 doses of hydroxychloroquine into its stockpile and we are making more. The threat of death is reduced substantially by this drug. When we go back to work, if doctors and the government advocate a prophylaxis of hydroxychloroquine or a cure in case of infection, all of America can go back to work with minimal risk. Don't you think the people in your circulation area of northeastern PA should know about this. Please.

Hospital workers, EMS/EMT workers, Police, Fire. warehouse workers, cashiers, manufacturing workers, etc. -- everybody can be safe rather than sorry.

-- End of 2nd email --

My two favorite antiviral drugs

1. Hydroxychloroquine
2. Remdesivir

[This was a year before Ivermectin came on the scene.

An existing, easy-to-produce medicine that proved effective at treating or preventing SARS-CoV-2 infection would provide the fastest relief for patients and doctors. As noted, the early hope is on hydroxychloroquine and chloroquine, and many hospitals, including the University of California, San Francisco, and the University of Washington, include them in their treatment guidelines. This anti-viral is approved for uses but not as a general treatment for COVID-19. My opinion is that it should have full FDA approval but I am not a doctor. According to the reports, it has saved lives.

1. Hydroxychloroquine, aka **Plaquenil**

Some doctors are combining hydroxychloroquine with azithromycin, an antibiotic. Much of the published evidence comes from a very small French study and reports from China. Larger, more rigorous clinical trials are starting, but they will take time. Favipiravir, a flu drug shown in Japan, appeared beneficial in another small study. These medicines, especially the malaria drugs, which are being mass-produced, will be used by doctors on the front lines, but we will have to wait for evidence of whether they are benefitting patients and how much.

2. Remdesivir

Timeline: First data could come in April.

Remdesivir, an antiviral medicine that failed as an Ebola treatment, was initially developed to work against a different coronavirus. There's some evidence that it benefits Covid-19 patients. Its maker, Gilead, has been working with researchers and governments around the world to get clinical trials up and running.

The company has said to expect results in April. Six large studies are in progress, with the first, in severely ill patients in China. It was due to finish as early as April 3, according to a government website.

A study in patients with milder disease will also finish in April, with two more due in May. In the meantime, Gilead has made the drug available to hundreds of patients on a compassionate use basis.

However, it recently said that, due to overwhelming demand, it would suspend access to the drug for all but pregnant women and children as it works to create a more systematic way of giving it out without interfering with clinical trials. This new system should be in place soon. Remdesivir must be given intravenously.

University of Minnesota tests all-in for hydroxychloroquine

Each day, other than supply, it looks better for hydroxychloroquine. It is getting lots of attention by lots of epidemiologists and the University of Minnesota.

At least three clinical trials for hydroxychloroquine are trying to establish whether the decades-old malaria medication can prevent COVID-19 infections in frontline health-care workers as hospitals across the country scramble to secure enough gowns and masks for their employees.

This includes two clinical trials at the University of Minnesota testing hydroxychloroquine in health care workers reporting pre- and post-exposure to the novel coronavirus. A third trial, funded by a government agency, wants to know if the drug can prevent infections in 15,000 health care workers. See my letter to the editor earlier in this section.

There is growing concern that the current strain on the health care system and its workers isn't sustainable given the high rates of exposure faced by clinicians working in frontline emergency rooms, intensive care units, and newly established COVID-19 units. At the same time, clinicians are being asked to wear one mask per shift or reuse them at some hospitals.

The COVID-19 pandemic has sickened more than 1 million people worldwide, including over 600,000 in the U.S. Over 32,000 people have died in the US. In the U.S., more and more clinicians are contracting the virus, and some are dying.

"The lack of workplace and patient safety right now is catastrophic," Rebecca Givan, an associate professor of labor studies and employment relations at Rutgers University, said in an email.

"Hospitals need to be honest with their workers, and do everything in their power to keep workers safe so that they can continue to provide desperately needed patient care without jeopardizing their own health or that of their families." Hydroxychloroquine can save their employee's lives.

Serological testing for antibodies

A week ago when Trump announced that Peter Navarro had procured over 29 million doses of hydroxychloroquine for the storehouse, the drug began to surge out of the storehouses and into pharmacies across the country. Now, just like there is a shortage of COVID-10 testing and serological testing supplies and the ability to get readouts, there will soon be a shortage of this powerful anti-viral drug and so the stockpile needs to be replaced. It is my opinion that hydroxychloroquine is vital to the success of an American economic restart.

This note is from the Commissioner of Food and Drugs, Food and Drug Administration, Stephen M. Hahn M.D. It explains the tests for antibodies which many believe will play a role in reopening America. Here is the commissioner's note:

> Serological tests measure the amount of antibodies or proteins present in the blood when the body is responding to a specific infection, like COVID-19. In other words, the test detects the body's immune response to the infection caused by the virus rather than detecting the virus itself. In the early days of an infection when the body's immune response is still building, antibodies may not be detected. This limits the test's effectiveness for diagnosing COVID-19 and why it should not be used as the sole basis to diagnose COVID-19.
>
> Serological tests can play a critical role in the fight against COVID-19 by helping healthcare professionals to identify individuals who have overcome an infection in the past and have developed an immune response. In the future, this may potentially be used to help determine, together with other clinical data, that such individuals are no longer susceptible to infection and can return to work. In addition, these test results can aid in determining who may donate a part of their blood called convalescent plasma, which may serve as a possible treatment for those who are seriously ill from COVID-19. This is why Vice President Mike Pence called on the laboratory community to develop serological tests for COVID-19.
>
> In March, the FDA issued a policy to allow developers of certain serological tests to begin to market or use their tests once they have performed the appropriate

evaluation to determine that their tests are accurate and reliable. This includes allowing developers to market their tests without prior FDA review if certain conditions outlined in the guidance document are met. The FDA issued this policy to allow early patient access to certain serological tests with the understanding that the FDA has not reviewed and authorized them.

The FDA can also authorize tests for COVID-19 under an Emergency Use Authorization (EUA). To date, FDA has authorized one EUA for a serological test that is intended for use by clinical laboratories.

Since the FDA issued the policy, over 70 test developers have notified the agency that they have serological tests available for use. However, some firms are falsely claiming that their serological tests are FDA approved or authorized, or falsely claiming that they can diagnose COVID-19. The FDA will take appropriate action against firms making false claims or marketing tests that are not accurate and reliable.

The FDA, an agency within the U.S. Department of Health and Human Services, protects the public health by assuring the safety, effectiveness, and security of human and veterinary drugs, vaccines and other biological products for human use, and medical devices. The agency also is responsible for the safety and security of our nation's food supply, cosmetics, dietary supplements, products that give off electronic radiation, and for regulating tobacco products.

How do we open up America?

One of the approaches to opening up America has to do with seeing who has had the virus in the past so that they can gain a certification to prove that person cannot be infected again. If there were an adequate supply of the antibody tests, this would be difficult to implement on a good day.

The notion of having to prove you're OK to get your freedom to work and walk around certificate may not fly well in a free country. That can be an obstacle as the day gets closer that we open up the country. I think we need a simpler approach. Serology testing may make us feel that we are OK but proving it to an employer or anybody else is going to be problematic. There are after all, 330 million citizens in just America to worry about. There are 7.8 billion worldwide.

There was a headline today that certainly got my attention. It said:

DON'T COUNT ON ANTIBODY TESTS TO REOPEN AMERICA

It offered that blood tests that measure a person's antibodies to the coronavirus could be a powerful tool to determine when it's safe to reopen the country. That is correct.

But after all the good news about the creation and development of such tests, concerns now exist about the accuracy and availability of the tests. Here is how the tests work:

Like the FDA Commissioner said: They detect whether a person has ever been exposed to the virus. But, there are many different tests than the single FDA approved test. These tests are different from those used to diagnose the disease. There are those who believe the existence of all these tests could hamper plans to allow Americans back to work and school.

Entrepreneurial America has created more than 90 different antibody tests. They are all now on the market, but only one has been authorized by the Food and Drug Administration. Why is this? The others "may not be as accurate as we'd like," agency FDA chief Stephen Hahn said recently as talk is ramping up about lifting the shutdown. Hahn's FDA has not verified the other 90 tests as being effective. Surely John Q. Public is not qualified to make this determination.

Public health experts are now warning that just because a person has antibodies to the coronavirus does not necessarily mean that they are immune to the virus, according to David Lim ...... But the antibody testing push comes as President Donald Trump is laser-focused on reopening the economy and governors on both coasts work on plans for a regional restart.

Rhode Island Gov. Gina Raimondo said her administration is already conducting a "deep dive, industry by industry" for guidelines to a "new normal,"

My personal concern is that government can easily guess wrong on who can do what and when in any piecemeal approach to relieving the shutdown. Unlike Dr. Fauci, I advocate turning the switch so we do not have to designate a ***grand determinator*** at the federal or state level to determine what are the gauntlet points that must be accomplished for a person to be declared free of disease, and then what? ?

So, what do we do about new screening and training for businesses that reopen. What must employees do to qualify? Where do they go? Pennsylvania for example has no testing facilities as of today—no drive throughs. Governor Raimondo is one of six northeast governors working together in a new working group announced Monday. There is a lot of hope for this group but there are a lot of pitfalls. Who makes the decisions for the group if they are independent of the president.

"Everyone is very anxious to get out of the house, get back to work, get the economy moving. Everyone agrees with that," said New York Gov. Andrew Cuomo. "What the art form is going to be here is doing that smartly, and doing that productively, and doing that in a coordinated way."

My perspective is to not put a whole load of *gotchas* and *have-tos* and, on the public or businesses. I say" "Let it happen naturally. "The people such as myself and my wife are going to be cautious entering this new open world. Let it up to us make those decisions as to what, and how. The government should just say when!

We got into this mess because it was unexpected. Nobody knew the risks of droplets or dirty hands or close contact. We have seen the case counts, and the deaths. Only a fool would act haphazardly if the switch were turned back on for the economy to start a of a certain date.

The governors' announcement came yesterday as the President asserted that he, not they, would decide when stay-at-home orders could be lifted. It also coincided with news from California Gov. Gavin Newsom, Oregon Gov. Kate Brown and Washington Gov. Jay Inslee that they are working on their own "shared approach" to restarting the West Coast economy and it does not depend on what the East Coast does.

Trump, as expected was asked about the governors' efforts during the Monday Task Force press briefing. Trump was emphatic: "a president's authority is ***total***." He added, "And that's the way it's got to be… And the governors know that." Legal scholars say the federal government lacks the power to directly order states to reopen their economies. The last thing America needs is a Constitutional fight before we can open America.

The simplest formula to open the country

Today is April 16, 2020. If I were in charge of the reopening of America, this would be the recommended approach:

It is based on every person's having a desire to survive.

1. All employees preparing to go back to work or already working or those people planning to not stay in 100% lockdown should see their doctor or clinician first; discuss their plans; schedule a test, and if you do not have antibodies, get a prescription for the hydroxychloroquine prophylaxis.

2. States need to designate areas for serology and disease testing and medicine dispensing. I know that I would not know where to go if the tests were ready tomorrow. Hydroxychloroquine prophylaxis needs to be made available as the prime solution. Patients should be able to get their dosage at:

   A. Doctors' Offices
   B. Clinics
   C. Private Urgent Care facilities
   D. Additional Facilities such as pharmacies and private areas staffed by PAs and / or nurses.
   E. Doctor. Med professional recommended prophylaxis should be taken by all workers who feel the need to wear masks.

3. Shutdown is lifted across the country on May 4 to May 11, 2020

4. Behavioral recommendations (not mandatory) are continued

Social distancing, hand washing etc. Avoid contact if not necessary. A new rule book of how to stay safe should be put together and made available

5. All businesses, entertainment, including restaurants, plays, movies, gymnasiums, swimming pools, parks, etc. may open. People need to voluntarily exercise caution like during the shutdown to avoid crowds if possible. If a place is crowded, go someplace else. If you are sick, stay home

6. Mass transportation reopens. Transit workers take prophylaxis.

7. Face masks recommended until further notice but not mandatory

8. People should stay at home except when they decide to go out to movies or dinner, etc. No restrictions on visiting neighbors or family other than in hospitals and nursing homes.

9. Employees will be called back to work by employers. They have five days to report to work. Those fearful to return to work may request up to 30 days additional leave. Unemployment compensation available for the thirty days for those called back to work – perhaps at half rate.

Summary

In early 2020, in retrospect, we did not know too much and we were all guessing.

Instead of the government determining what is best for the people, the people have already suffered for more than four weeks with the country in lockdown, and the people understand the risks by now. The people are naturally cautious and restrictions will not make us more cautious.

Over time, we may choose to brave the outside world when we feel the time is right. Plus, we may opt to dine inside a restaurant with or without a prophylaxis such as hydroxychloroquine. The medicine which would serve as a crutch so that we would not be infected. Use similar cautions to now to protect yourself from infection.

I would recommend taking the proper amount of a prophylaxis such as hydroxychloroquine to ward off the virus. This medicine may last about three weeks or perhaps longer. Renew the prophylaxis regimen as required. This would be more effective than the antibodies testing and the drug can be made more available than the test. The idea is that eventually the coronavirus will be gone.

If you think you have contracted the virus or are concerned about it, you should get tested wherever you can. If positive, ask the physician or attendant for a prescription for hydroxychloroquine with a packet of Zinc and another prescription for Azithromycin. This "three pack" has been effective in curing the virus in some people. It can cure the virus but it is not 100% guaranteed.

Go home and quarantine for 14 days while taking the medicine until the doctor says you no longer have the virus. If you do not improve, call your doctor. Like all medicine, nothing is 100% but hydroxychloroquine is one that I would be looking for if I get sick.

It should be part of the nation's recommended solution for reopening.

By all means reopen the country so we have an economy ready to go when we as a country are finally ready to stop hibernating.

CHAPTER 8

Was the FDA's Hydroxy Decision based on Politics?

You bet it was! What a shame!.

This chapter has its basis in a number of facts that I collected from the Stats article by Nicholas Fiorko on June 16, 2020 titled: *What does the FDA's hydroxychloroquine decision mean for Covid-19 patients or politicians?* Great article but the FDA should be ashamed of itself. It is over two years old but still hits the mark.

This is the fifth year and there is still plenty of Trump hate to go around. The hydroxychloroquine controversy was not a controversy at all until Trump said something good about the medicine. When Trump said something positive about hydroxychloroquine, it was the kiss of death for the medication. Hard to believe but true, nonetheless. America was affected by the Left's disinformation campaign.

The Never Trumpers and the Trump Haters went to work immediately to punish a hitherto malaria drug and Lupus drug even using face trials and fake stories about it affecting the rhythm of the heart in COVID patients. Get this: Somehow it was OK according to the FDA for malaria prophylaxis and for curing malaria and it was OK to fight the storms prevalent in Lupus infections. No problemo.

That was about the time in the pandemic that the people began to notice the politization of our most prestigious health agencies the FDA, the CDC, and the NIH. Wanting to stay on the good side of the progressives and the liberals and the Marxists, the FDA wasted no time in letting the Democrats know they controlled the FDA even though Trump was still president. They more or less apologized for going against the leftists by having granted an emergency use authorization for hydroxychloroquine at the urgings of then President Donald Trump.

On June 16, 2020 after just a few months of permitting temporary use of hydroxychloroquine for COVID patients, under severe Democrat pressure, the Food & Drug Administration relented and acceded to the demands of the Trump haters. These *no-minds* had instantly become hydroxychloroquine haters as if by punishing the drug and those who liked it, vicariously they would be punishing Trump.

So in a major act of appeasement, the FDA revoked its already controversial emergency use decision for the malaria drug hydroxychloroquine— an eyebrow-raising reversal that had sweeping implications for how America could respond to Covid-19.

The decision, which flew in the face of President Trump's own touting of the medicine as a treatment for Covid-19, was more than just a stunning rebuke of a president by his own administration though that was the real intent. In fact, the decision was likely to and in fact did hurt a lot of people from governors who scrambled to assemble stockpiles of the drug for their states, to patients asking their family physician for a chance to try the drug. Shame on the FDA for not defending Americans and America.

During this period, it certainly appeared that whenever a clinical trial demonstrated efficacy it somehow did not become one of the valid reliable test cases. Why was that? Politics! In June 2020, when the FDA canceled hydroxychloroquine, there were still over 100 active and recruiting clinical trials. They were in place to test hydroxychloroquine as a treatment for the disease caused by the novel coronavirus.

The FDA simply could not wait to see the results. Instead they wanted the trials to fail because of the politics and the power of the Democrat Party.

When they made the proclamation that the drug is "unlikely to be effective in treating Covid-19, and that it could be dangerous to healthy Americans it was clear to most that they were blowing smoke as the medicine had already been used effectively for malaria for 65 years and had recently become the go-to medicine (Plaquenil) recently for Lupus patients. Besides this, the FDA created another reason—"serious side effects." Somehow those side effects did not affect the use of the medicine for malaria and Lupus. How is that? That does not make sense. Either it has side affects or it does not—independent of its use.

What did the FDA's decision actually mean? Well, the FDA would have been better off saying nothing. It was supposed to mean that the FDA theoretically lost confidence that hydroxychloroquine was an effective treatment for Covid-19. To me and millions of other Americans it meant that the Democrats had finally succeeded in politicizing the nation's top medicine authority and the FDA lost its credibility with many, many Americans from that moment on.

One concern about the FDA's politically-motivated decision is that it might make hospitals, doctors, patients and families really think twice. That's what the Democrats wanted as a way of showing Trump that he was not the boss.

The US policy all of a sudden meant that the Strategic National Stockpile would no longer distribute doses of hydroxychloroquine and chloroquine to hospitalized patients being treated for Covid-19. I would like to see the study that follows about how many people succumb who would have otherwise lived.

Hospitals had been encouraged this time and still are by Democrats and now the FDA to wind down using any of those drugs that they have left on hand for Covid-19 patients. In an FDA frequently-asked-questions document, the agency said that hospitals who have already begun treating existing patients with hydroxychloroquine provided from the stockpile could continue doing so, but that treating new patients with these drugs is no longer "authorized." Amazing!

Here is the rationale spoken directly by the FDA. Basically anybody that does not follow their guidance does so at their own risk.

Welcome to the FDA Drug Safety Podcast for health care professionals.

On April 24, 2020 FDA announced that we are aware of reports of serious heart rhythm problems in patients with COVID-19 treated with hydroxychloroquine or chloroquine, often in combination with azithromycin and other QT prolonging medicines. We are also aware of increased use of these medicines through outpatient prescriptions. We are reminding health care professionals and patients of the known risks associated with both hydroxychloroquine and chloroquine.

Hydroxychloroquine and chloroquine have not been shown to be safe and effective for treating or preventing COVID-19. They are being studied in clinical trials for COVID-19, and we authorized their temporary use during the COVID-19 pandemic for treatment of the virus in hospitalized patients when clinical trials are not available, or participation is not feasible, through an Emergency Use Authorization (or EUA). The medicines being used under this EUA are supplied from the Strategic National Stockpile, the national repository of critical medical supplies to be used during public health emergencies. This safety communication reminds physicians and the public of risk information set out in the hydroxychloroquine and chloroquine healthcare provider fact sheets that were required by the EUA.

Hydroxychloroquine and chloroquine can cause abnormal heart rhythms such as QT interval prolongation and ventricular tachycardia. These risks may increase when these medicines are combined with other medicines known to prolong the QT interval, including azithromycin.

We are warning the public that hydroxychloroquine and chloroquine, either alone or combined with azithromycin, when used for COVID-19 should be limited to clinical trial settings or for treating certain hospitalized patients under the EUA.

Hydroxychloroquine and chloroquine are FDA-approved to treat or prevent malaria. Hydroxychloroquine is also FDA-approved to treat autoimmune conditions such as chronic discoid lupus erythematosus, systemic lupus erythematosus in adults, and rheumatoid arthritis.

The EUA was based upon limited evidence that the medicines may provide benefit, and for this reason, we authorized their use only in hospitalized patients under careful heart monitoring. If a healthcare professional is considering use of hydroxychloroquine or chloroquine to treat or prevent COVID-19, FDA recommends checking www.clinicaltrials.gov for a suitable clinical trial and consider enrolling the patient...

It remains to be determined, however, how the FDA was able to force hospitals to not begin new patients on these drugs. How does the drug itself differentiate whether it is from a stockpile or it was recently delivered? Strange. Too strange perhaps for it to be the truth.

One thing for sure. Hydroxychloroquine has not completely gone away. Yes, the old stand-by Hydroxychloroquine, the antimalarial drug that former President Donald Trump touted as a "game changer" in the fight against Covid-19, is still being prescribed by physicians in the U.S. though, according to the skeptics and the FDA, it has proven to be ineffective against the virus in clinical trials. Despite this evidence, persistent physicians suggest there has never been a trial in which there was not bias and nobody has their reputation on the line about its being a success or failure.

Concern had been growing by skeptics that patients are at risk of harm because stubborn physicians continue to prescribe hydroxychloroquine over other potentially life-saving COVID treatments. In June, 2020, we know the Food and Drug Administration (FDA) revoked the emergency use authorization (EUA) for hydroxychloroquine "in light of ongoing serious cardiac adverse events and other serious side effects." The FDA suggests that the potential benefits of the drug no longer outweigh the known and potential risks for the authorized use, the agency said in a statement.

The bottom line is Democrats won and Conservative Americans lost in being able to use one of the most effective COVID fighters in the arsenal according to my own research. And, I admit that I am not a doctor but neither am I influenced by political reasoning for medical decisions. What a shame for America.

A would-be chain of cancer centers now wants to treat patients with Right to Try drugs, raising ethical questions.

My state has its own stockpile, what happens to that?

As expected states that stocked up were annoyed at the FDA like the rest of us. More than 20 states have created their own stockpiles of hydroxychloroquine. Those states immediately went to limbo.

Technically speaking, there were not any legal reason for states to abandon their stockpiles, so long as they relied on donations of FDA-approved versions of these drugs or purchased FDA-approved versions of the drugs directly from manufacturers.

It remains to be seen, however, whether states will still want to stand behind hydroxychloroquine. STAT reached out to nearly a dozen states for comment on the FDA's decision. A spokesperson for North Carolina told STAT that the state is making an assessment about what to do with the supplies that they have on hand." Spokespeople for Texas and New York said similar feelings, but noted that their states have not distributed any doses from their stockpiles since late April. And a spokesperson for Louisiana said it is contacting manufacturers to see if they can send the drug back. The bottom line is their responses are all hooey.

Can a patient who wants to take hydroxychloroquine still take it?

Yes, so long as they can find a doctor who will write them a prescription. Depending on the politics of the doctorand the pharmacy, you may be OK. The FDA does not police so-called off-label prescribing, where a doctor uses an FDA-approved drug to treat a condition such as malaria even though the intended use might be COVID-19.

So, hydroxychloroquine is approved to treat malaria and lupus. Therefore doctors can use it to treat any condition they want, including Covid-19. The FDA's decision to revoke this authorization has no impact on that and it should not. Consequently other than bragging rights for Democrats, withdrawing the emergency use authorization may have relatively little practical impact. That is because of the fact that doctors can still prescribe hydroxychloroquine off-label.

This seems like it could be a political nightmare for Republicans.

Democrats certainly hope so.

We know that Democrat-induced-agencies are against everything but big Pharma vaccinations. Yet there are still a lot of physicians who do not buy into their babble. I read an article recently about two such men, who "want you to think that ivermectin could be all we need to treat, or even prevent, any COVID-19 case." They are Dr. Pierre Kory, a former critical-care specialist at the University of Wisconsin medical center, and Dr. Paul Marik, the chief of critical care at Eastern Virginia Medical School. I would bet their patients love them.

Together, Kory and Marik lead the Front Line COVID-19 Critical Care Alliance, a nonprofit organization founded by "fringe doctors" and former media pros that has led an increasingly concerted campaign, hinged on "twisted science," to promote ivermectin as a cure-all for COVID-19. You can see the palpable bias in the way the article was written.

Here is some more babble: "Ivermectin is effectively a 'miracle drug' against COVID-19," Kory told members of the Senate homeland-security committee last December, saying data showed profound efficacy" of the drug "in all stages of the disease."

He concluded that if everyone were to have access to the antiparasitic, "the pandemic will end, the economy can reopen, social interactions and activity can resume, and life can normalize."

How is that for an endorsement. The religion against hydroxychloroquine and Invermectin is winning the battle but not necessarily because of truth, justice, and the American way.

We know that in the last election cycle Hydroxychloroquine became a focal point in a number of congressional races, with Democrats criticizing several Republican lawmakers and hopefuls for being enthusiastic about the medicine before there was evidence to support it as a treatment for Covid-19. The FDA decision of course will bolster that criticism.

To show the politics of the matter, the Democratic Congressional Campaign Committee has issued press releases slamming Republican congressional candidates who have been targeted by the Democrats for supporting Hydroxychloroquine. This should have nothing to do with politics, but tell a Democrat that and see how far you get.

Congressional Democrats pounced on the president after the FDA announcement: Is this politics or what? They announced: "America: do not listen to President Trump on any medical advice. His own FDA is rejecting his advice on Hydroxychloroquine," Senate Minority Leader Chuck Schumer of New York tweeted. Ask yourself "do you believe Marist Senator Chuck Schumer speaks for America?

There were immediate signs that FDA warnings would not be enough to convince voters that Hydroxychloroquine doesn't work. A May poll from Morning Consult and Politico found that 24% of voters strongly supported or somewhat supported use of the drug, despite the FDA's warnings that it shouldn't be used outside of a clinical trial. Another 31% were unsure.

What's at stake for industry in the pharmaceutical Space Race for a Covid-19 vaccine

Is hydroxychloroquine-mania over? Considering that a year later, with the broad introduction of Ivermectin for COVOD-19, the question could be asked about both of these "wonder drugs."

Interest in the drugs could also grow again as more clinical trials readout. There are still over 100 active or recruiting clinical trials testing hydroxychloroquine for example, as a Covid-19 treatment, according to clinicaltrials.gov. The FDA's decision has no impact on those clinical trials, and if one or more have positive results, that will almost definitely reignite interest over this effective medicine.

Remember folks, it is not nice and can be an uphill battle to fight mother nature in the form of the FDA or any and all government agencies trying to convince them to change their stance on COVID. We have all seen how Democrat causes from mask mandates, required vaccinations, Critical Race Theory, Anti First & Second Amendment, no drilling, high inflation etc. Try arguing with any of them and you will ruin your day. COVID is in the same religious lessons.

The HCQ debate is far from over & not one the liberal media here in the US can silence. The simple fact is that the trials that have been referenced for discrediting its use to reduce saturation of COVID-19 in the lungs have not followed anywhere close to guidelines defined in the anecdotal reports of its successful usage. Those reports from nations like France led to massive petition drives (100-500K signatures) in many nations lobbying their governments to make HCQ readily available for COVID-19 treatment.

What's worse is that the trials in question for discrediting HCQ treatment of COVID-19 saturation in the lungs have used what many consider "lethal" doses of the drug. They rigged the trials and may have killed patients. Pres Trump was taking just 200mg of HCQ & other combinates to prevent the saturation of COVID-19 in his lungs should he become infected with SARS-V2. These trials used over 2000mg of HCQ daily. I'm not aware of a single anecdotal report of successful usage of HCQ using anywhere close to that dosage. What was their purpose – assured failure? Is there any truth left in America?

That is medical malpractice & a waiver is not going to protect the parties involved. When the families of the dead in these trials learn about these lethal doses there will be protests & calls for class action lawsuits against the physicians that conducted them.

Fiorko notes that "Liberals were caught with their pants down over the Brexit movement & this HCQ movement is showing similar signs". While the FDA has discredited the medicine mainly based on trial data where lethal doses & other irresponsible behavior occurred, both the number of clinical trials & stockpiles continue to grow. The people demand hydrochloroquine and the doctors know it.

This has the potential to devastate the DNC & other parts of the liberal establishment world over both now & in the near future. If I were them I would at least leave the door open as to the promise of HCQ vs COVID-19 in the lungs when used RESPONSIBLY. Lethal doses result in lethal results.

On June 16, Andrej commented on FIorko's article

Any good scientist, who has no political leaning, knows that HCQ works.

1. It is an antiviral and an ionophore
2. Needs to be given early.
3. Needs to be given with Zinc
4. Azithro may be given as well to boost effectiveness

Poorly designed studies have been published, with some even being retracted from prestigious journals, whose only aim is to try and discredit HCQ.

These are all scientific hacks, who should be ashamed to be grouped with good scientists and medical professionals.

HCQ has been a safe drug for 65 years and perhaps even 85 years. It has been readily prescribed to pregnant women. It has less adverse event reports than Tylenol or aspirin.

Sad, sad time for science. Being dragged through the mud by special interest political groups.

On June 16, Dr. James commented on FIorko's article

The clinical jury is still out on HCQ, notwithstanding the studies referenced here. For example, India loves it, as do the GCC states. Both are doing far better than New York (for example) where HCQ was essentially banned for outpatient use by Cuomo's 23 March exec order. To date no reliable studies show it is harmful. So if it turns out that HCQ is effective, it's FDA that will look like a complete ass, along with all the blue anti-HCQ crowd. OTOH, if HCQ turns out to be totally useless, go blue! Get out the popcorn.

On June 16, Dean commented on Florko's article

Thank you Dr. John for your wealth of information via the many links to experts in your comments. You certainly filled in for what STAT failed to do: share smart, well-resourced expert info. Instead, STAT again writes politics infused babble, which is highly annoying, not informative, and just as low as the presented lobs at the biased uninformed President. So thank you, Dr. Abeles, for your input !!

On June 18, Dr. John commented on Florko's article

Thanks for the kind words

The persistent, almost gleeful, denigration of a promising oral antiviral combination therapy in EARLY SARS-CoV-2 infection i.e. for the large number of outpatients – in the shape of a regimen of hydroxychloroquine plus added other drugs – because of equivocal results in LATE therapy in hospitalized patients (who could be said to have a different disease syndrome than non-hospitalized patients) and without the added co-drugs in the regimen – most notably adequate, added zinc as many people have zinc store deficiencies – is a mounting tragedy and unparalleled in my long experience

It does smack of political motivation to my mind which is a great pity.

Hopefully there are well designed, prospective, controlled studies ongoing to fully test in early Covid19 outpatients the substantial, positive, preclinical and observational, large-scale case reports to date plus some smaller double blind controlled studies as well ...

One of the best reviews on the matter is from Dr Hirsch of Yale University – it can be read here :

https://academic.oup.com/aje/advance-article/doi/10.1093/aje/kwaa093/5847586

On June 17, Lisa Hall commented on FIorko's article

This drug DOES work and there have been hundreds of patients in the US alone who were very sick with COVID and within 2 days they were remarkably better. So, for the FDA to come out with this statement is such a political move by the Liberals; shame on the FDA for playing the politics game. Very disappointed in you.

CHAPTER 9

Comments on the Goodness of Hydroxychloroquine

Fox News's Laura Ingraham has been fighting the COVID battle from the beginning. She does not buy the bull the left and their three US agency surrogates are throwing. To put the story to rest Laura already said she would be willing to volunteer to test whether hydroxychloroquine, a drug used on malaria and arthritis patients, could help with the Coronavirus.

Ingraham on her show said that it would take a controlled 2,000-patient study and that such a study "could be organized pretty quickly" given the high stakes meaning of the results. Let's do it! Let's get at the truth.

At the time of her pronouncement, Laura said: "I have a feeling given the fact that most of the countries are locked down right now, the controlled study of 2,000 patients could be organized pretty quickly, given what is at stake here, "I'll happily volunteer. If you're looking for volunteers, I'll volunteer."

Two members of the *multi-year medicine cabinet* formed by Laura Ingraham, Drs. Ramin Oskoui, cardiologist and CEO of Foxhall cardiology, and Stephen Smith, founder of the Smith Center for

Infectious Diseases and Urban Health, often join Laura Ingraham on her Fox show "The Ingraham Angle." These two doctors have the goods on the Hydroxychloroquine controversy as they have been prescribing it with great results on patients who the CDC, NIH, and FDA would choose to leave to die.

Ingraham says there is no truthful Democrat leadership, and they are wrong on every front, especially therapeutics such as hydroxychloroquine. Ingraham asks "How can Democrats govern a country that they hate?" Think about that question for awhile folks and their reaction to saving Americans with Hydroxychloroquine is more understandable.

Here is some text from a recent show. Parts of this are from a rush transcript from "The Ingraham Angle. Not all of the show is in this chapter—just enough to give you the right perspective. Our thanks to Laura for this contribution. Watch the show. It is well worth your time:

INGRAHAM: All right. I'm Laura Ingraham. This is THE INGRAHAM ANGLE from Washington tonight. We have a lot to get to. An original member of our medicine cabinet is here with new and exhaustive analysis of hydroxychloroquine. We're going to share it with you.

STEPHEN SMITH, SMITH CENTER FOR INFECTIOUS DISEASES: Infectious doctors are not familiar with Hydroxychloroquine, which is not a traditional antibiotic. It affects the host cell metabolism. And I know it's effective, so I'm not going to say, I think, it's effective. I know it is from our data.

INGRAHAM: We have that data over a year later that Dr. Stephen Smith promised. In a new study, Smith and three other medical experts prove what he and this show have been telling you for more than a year that hydroxychloroquine can save lives.

Smith's landmark study followed 255 COVID patients who required intubation during the first two months of the pandemic. And it found that increased doses of co-administered hydroxychloroquine and azithromycin were associated with a greater than 100 percent increase in survival. Here now Dr. Stephen Smith, Founder of the Smith Center for Infectious Diseases and Urban Health. Dr. Smith, why were so many people so quick to dismiss what you were seeing with your own eyes, your own experience early on?

SMITH: There's a lot of fear. I mean, obviously there was strange political reasons that I'll never understand. Again, back to those comments, infectious disease doctors who in charge of deciding how much hydroxychloroquine to give and for how long, the early reports of how much to give were very low.

There are suggestions, based off of pharmacokinetic studies - very, very low. 2,400 milligrams over five days. And I turned to the pharmacist, Steve Smoke at St. Barnabas and I said, I got people that are literally more than four times difference in weight, one or both groups is getting the wrong dose.

And so I started reading it and then of course, Dr. (inaudible) and colleagues came out with their regimen which is still not a high dose. I would say higher dose because it's not a high dose of hydroxychloroquine. Its 6,000 milligrams every 10 days, that's nothing compared to what any lupus patient or any rheumatoid arthritis patient takes.

Because they - one, that daily dose is not particularly high. But, two, more importantly, the drug builds up for 200 days. So you're taking 400 a day, which is, I would say a lower dose, you pass 600 - 6000 weight (ph) by 20 days easily and you keep going up higher—

INGRAHAM: But Dr. Smith, I mean, people watching they don't understand the dosage. I mean, that's very in the weeds, but it's critical, obviously. But today, tonight, are you able to use hydroxychloroquine with any COVID patients that may still be coming in?

SMITH: No. The hospital where we see patients St. Barnabas Medical Center in Livingston, I guess, the system wide thing we have several hospitals - they banned use of hydroxychloroquine in December for an indication. Meaning, if you're going to use it for COVID.

You can put anyone on hydroxychloroquine, if you think they have lupus, that's fine. If I - even if I decided I thought hydroxychloroquine worked just to treat migraines, I could use it for that too. That was a unique ban in American medicine, where they banned a drug by indication.

INGRAHAM: Now, how many lives do you think could have been saved had people had an open mind about hydroxychloroquine?

SMITH: Yes, I struggle with that when I tried really start to think about it. Our numbers were staggering. They're really not our numbers. They're - the only - this cohort of 255 patients required ventilation intubation only - 20 percent are mine, or our, my team's. So these results reflect the entire group, the whole hospital's results and--

INGRAHAM: OK. Well, we lost 500,000 patients. We lost over 500,000 Americans - 550,000 Americans. I mean, are we talking we could have saved 10,000 lives?

SMITH: No more than that, ma'am, a lot more.

INGRAHAM: 100,000?

SMITH: Yes. I - Laura, I hate to say things like that. But, yes, I mean, the data - you know, I just try and look at the data and these data - the study was not really just Hydroxychloroquine study by any means.

We looked at everything. We looked at every medicine ever given, every lab value, every vital sign. We looked at prior visits to doctors. But hydroxychloroquine kept coming up and it was it was a cumulative dose that was associated with outcome, not just whether you got some hydroxychloroquine like some of the studies.

INGRAHAM: This - I mean, this is out - I mean, outrageous. Doesn't begin to describe this. Criminal - I don't even think captures it what has happened here. But Dr. Smith, you have been consistent throughout and we just appreciate it so much. And we're going to, obviously have you back on all the other topics.

End of INGRAHAM show transcript.

This makes me sick. For political reasons people are dying and doctors cannot override hospital rules. Thank you Democrats. You must hate America and all Americans too.

Thanks a lot.

CHAPTER 10

Some HCQ Anecdotal Evidence

Many Americans have lost faith in our public-paid scientists such as Dr. Anthony Fauci because, quite frankly, they speak out of both sides of their mouths and different verbiage comes out from each side. Most Americans did not know until recently how lucrative it is to be in Fauci's National Spot. It was just reported that during the Pandemic, Dr. Fauci's net worth increased by over $5 million. It is now almost $13 million.

Americans don't care about the money but they do care about the truth. They feel the experts are either lying or incompetent or both. That's how I see it and it is how many Americans now view the "official word."

Until COVID-19 and the pandemic most of these useful idiots were in labs or cellars some place and did not surface often and the people could care about their existence. If we were asked about their importance in the US, without knowing anything most Americans would have given them glowing reports. CDC, NIF, FDA, etc. are big names in medical science and they supposedly are the stop-gap groups to assure that slippery characters do not unleash things that are bad for the health of Americans. But what if these respected icons of medicine are the slippery characters?

The perspective on them changed with COVID and the pandemic. Many of us now have Fauci-Fatigue from his changing principles—mask, no mask, mask, two-masks, three masks is even better etc. The eminent Fauci has been spewing whatever he thinks for the duration and he gets less believable the more he appears on CNN and MSNBC and other Democrat-controlled media outlets.

I do not know what they offer him but they sure treat him like he is the second coming. He seems to respond to their flattering with more pronouncements that fit their ideology. And, so, he and the rest of the public scientists become less and less believable.

The Democrats and all the Fauci's out there all say the same thing. And if you don't repeat what they say and you use your own mind, their friends in Big Tech will DE-platform you and take your first amendment rights to free speech away in a whisk.

My Democrat friends think this is OK because they speak in one voice. I have a lot of them and I know they get their news from CNN which is major spoke in the propaganda Cabal that controls what Democrats think. If CNN says something, they immediately believe it because somebody told them in their lives at some time that Republicans are bad and that Conservatives are bad and the only thing good is a Democrat.

I am a Democrat and have been all my life but when I ran for Congress and for Mayor in my home town I was defeated by those who were part of the Democrat machine and I was discredited for my views on life. I think for myself. My brothers and sisters think for themselves and my kids think for themselves. Most are hard and fast values oriented people who do not like the spew Democrats and their cohorts spread. To them and to me, when Democrats push an issue, I have gotten so cynical and so have they that there is a bigger reason than their personal opinion for their point of view.

Clearly not all Democrats are Woke but they will defend wokism to a fault. They are not all Marxists and now Communists but when their leaders spout Marxist and Communist principles, they buy-in 100%.. When I engage in discussions with them, it is obvious where they pick up their opinions. To them their opinions make them safe to be Democrats.

I expect this book to be censored by Amazon, the company I once used to print and distribute my books. I am my own publisher – Lets Go Publish! is my company. Letsgopublish.com is my web site. I never asked Amazon to read my books. They grabbed the power after buying out the competition and this past year they censored seventeen of my books and then they terminated my account and no longer sell my books.

Amazon does not like my ideology. We'll see soon if they let this book go out as it is. I speak my piece regardless as they control not just their own company's censoring but they extend their influence to other publishers.

Even if they do not choose to permit this book to be printed and distributed, you will be able to read it for free on Lets Go Publish! How is that? Because I will put it out for free. I may not make a dime but I won't be censored.

Amazon has a few pet authors that they permit books about the pandemic to write and they publish. Not me. I snuck one book out since Amazon decided it was my censor. For years, it wasavailable on Amazon and sold well. It's title is "Hydroxychloroquine: The Game Changer" I hoped Amazon lets this book alone, but they did not. They canceled it.

Anyway, I believe in hydroxychloroquine. If I get the bug, I want to take the medicine soon to get better—the sooner the better. I am vaccinated twice with Moderna. So I am not against being well. You think for yourself. But no more vaccinations for me. I think they are more dangerous to your health than is Hydroxychloroquine and Ivermectin.

I know you feel similarly or you would not be reading this book. As you read in the last chapter, Laura Ingraham says what the leftist Marxists, Communist Democrats have done to the ability for the public to get solid information about valid therapeutic "cures" for COVID is nothing less than CRIMINAL As a lawyer, I am sure Ingraham would love the opportunity to prosecute those who denied patients Hydroxychloroquine or Ivermectin. I would consider going to Law School if I could be assured of a crack at these fakes whose opinions have killed over a million people out of the over 100 million cases so far in the US.

I have a few stories about three people I know who take hydroxychloroquine regularly or who took it when they tested positive for COVID.

First please let me share with you some facts about chloroquine and hydroxychloroquine. In all I have researched however, I do not have a good explanation for why the medical community and all Democrats are against these two wonder drugs. I do think it is as simple as "Trump likes them." However, there is no truth to the besmirchment and the disdain, which they use to describe Chloroquine and Hydroxychloroquine. I picked the right word (besmirch) to describe what they do,

Well over sixty-five years ago, and perhaps as many as eighty-years, Chloroquine (CQ) was first used as prophylaxis and treatment for malaria. Hydroxychloroquine (HCQ) is a more soluble and less toxic metabolite of chloroquine, which causes less side effects and is, therefore, safer. We don't hear much about chloroquine since hydroxychloroquine is preferred and it is in ample supply.

In the past several years, CQ/HCQ has been used to manage conditions such as systemic lupus erythematosus and rheumatoid arthritis. You can't find a lupus patient or rheumatoid arthritis patient who does not take one of these, typically Hydroxychloroquine,

CQ/HCQ has also been used in the treatment of HIV with mixed results. Nobody in the medical field would have been prescribing Hydroxychloroquine for any of these maladies if it were harmful For sixty-five + years, it is the standard-bearer for malaria as a preventative (prophylaxis) and as a cure.

The ability of CQ/HCQ to inhibit certain coronaviruses, such as SARS-CoV-1, has been explored with promising results Both drugs are affordable and widely available internationally. With decades of experience administering these drugs, their safety profiles are well-established. It is likely to take many months for novel, specific treatments of COVID-19 to become available. As a result, there has been growing interest in the use of CQ and HCQ and Ivermectin as potential treatments in the interim. Of course these remedies for COVID would long ago have been approved if there was not so much bias against them because of political ideologies. What a shame.

Results from In Vitro and In Vivo Research

In Vitro Studies
There is preliminary in vitro evidence of the ability of CQ and HCQ to inhibit SARS-CoV-2 activity. In Vitro is experimentation without a patient – in the glass, if you will.

In Vivo Clinical Trials
The empirical evidence for the effectiveness of CQ/HCQ in COVID-19 is currently very limited. First clinical results were reported in a news briefing by the Chinese government in February 2020, revealing that the treatment of over 100 patients with chloroquine phosphate in China had resulted in significant improvements of pneumonia and lung imaging, with reductions in the duration of illness. No adverse events

were reported. It appears that these findings were a result of combining data from several ongoing trials using a variety of study designs. No empirical data supporting these findings have been published so far.

I asked a friend who had COVID to tell me about it before and after using hydroxychloroquine. This is anecdotal evidence that at least in this sample of 1, it sure did work.

Here is my request for information:

Brian Kelly Author Inquiry:

I need a favor. I do not want anything that is untrue but I am interested in knowing if you think hydroxychloroquine helped end your illness or not and by what degree. Were you taking anything else

Can you give me a timeline?
Take your time.
Thank you very much.
God bless. Stay well!

COVID Patient Response:

Sure, no problem. I can tell you about my experience as best as possible.

I felt really crappy on a Wednesday in April. I had just embarked on a new journey, going to a very intense gym every day starting that Monday. By the time Wednesday came around I was really sore and run down so I attributed that to my new gym venture. Then it was Saturday and my symptoms of fatigue and aches were rising... I was an 8 out of 10 on the feeling yucky scale. That's a scientific scale by the way...

I have had the flu a dozen times and to be perfectly honest that's exactly what it felt like. My fever never broke 100 but I was running 99.9ish when I finally went to the Med Express in Edwardsville that Saturday afternoon.

I asked if they could test me for the flu and the physician assistant snickered at me and said no sorry we only test for COVID. I said okay well last year I was diagnosed with influenza A right here in this clinic and I feel like I did then. She said I'll be right back with your COVID test.

After the PA swabbed my brain stem through my nostrils she left the room for a few minutes and came back in to tell me I was COVID+. I immediately asked her if she would Rx me hydroxychloroquine. She laughed and said I hope you are joking. She said stop listening to conspiracy theories that stuff does not treat COVID. I didn't argue with her beyond that because I only have a bachelor's degree and she went to med school so she must be way smarter than I am.

They sent me home with no treatment just said drink fluids.

I can't recall exactly when I received the HCQ dose. It was 1 or 2 days after my MedExpress appointment. I began the protocol immediately, taking HCQ 200mg 3x daily along with zinc and Z-pack. Within the next 48hrs I noticed marked improvement in my body aches and fatigue. Within 72hrs I would say that I had complete resolution of my symptoms. I continued to take the medication until there were no more pills left. I have been feeling great ever since I beat COVID, no return of symptoms whatsoever.

Today I was prescribed the Ivermectin prevention protocol by a local doctor. If you are interested in meeting this doctor or if you know anyone who may want to meet him he is more than willing to help others in our community.

If you have any questions or need anything else, let me know.

Have a great week!

Two Lupus Patients

I have two friends with Lupus. Both take Plaquenil, which is a brand name for hydroxychloroquine as prescribed for Lupus patients. One is about 60 years old and he is very healthy and the other is about 70 and she has had a number of medical issues besides Lupus.

Both of them are reasonably active but mask in places where they should mask and like most of us, they try to use social distancing during the pandemic. They are not hypochondriacs.

As I reported in this book, I have not ever read an article in which the author suggested that any Lupus patient had contracted COVID. Neither of my two friends contracted COVID so far. I think the fact that Lupus patients take hydroxychloroquine, they gain the prophylaxis (preventative) aspects of the medicine in addition to its fighting their Lupus flares for them. Obviously my sample is just two people but look it up yourself and tell me if there are any documented cases of a Lupus patient contracting COVID-19?

There is no reason on earth for medical scientists to block the use of hydroxychloroquine when the results in so many are so good. I agree with Laura Ingraham. What they have done by depriving the American people of a potential cure is criminal There are 100,000 souls in heaven who would still be living according to Dr. Smith. Remember that when somebody tells you it has been disproven. That' my friends is a bold-faced lie. It is definitely criminal

CHAPTER 11

That's Not All There Is

Just further proof that Hydroxychloroquine and Ivermectin have not reached the physicians most prescribed list for COVID, I have this true story. Within the last several weeks separated by a few weeks, my two wonderful sisters Nancy & Mary came down with the COVID-19 virus whichever version is most popular nowadays. Neither of my sisters were prescribed Hydroxychloroquine nor Ivermectin but that does not mean that they could not have.

As you know from this book so far, the flowing water containing the major success stories of Hydroxychloroquine and Invermectin are still muddy and murky. That does not mean that there are not thousands of physicians who are sold on the treatment and are devotees of prescribing these two therapeutics for COVID-19.

Two years ago I was convinced and now with even more remedies available I still believe in both therapeutics but I don't feel that either have caught on and quite frankly whereas a few years ago it was easy to believe in them, today even I would simply listen to my doctor.

I am not saying that if I tested positive and had either Hydroxychloroquine or Ivermectin on hand from a past legitimate prescription that I would not take it before I even called my doctor. That is not my recommendation but it is what I would do. I do believe that the best approach, however is to contact your doctor immediately upon testing positive if not sooner.

My sister Nancy for example is all better now and she was prescribed Paxlovid. My sister Mary is almost finished with her course of prescribed Lagevrio. She is lots better and has just a bit to go. With both of these, their respective doctors recommended they take Vitamin D, Vitamin C and Zinc. Even when Hydroxychloroquine and/or Invermectin were first on the list, the same course of vitamins and minerals was also recommended.

Pharmaceuticals often have pesudonyms or proper names and these two are the same. For example, The other names for Paxlovid are (nirmatrelvir/ritonavir) and the other name for Lagevrio is molnupiravir. These are two oral antiviral treatments that are authorized to treat mild to moderate COVID-19. These COVID-19 pills are only recommended for people with a high risk of developing severe illness.

Later in this chapter, when I discuss the Mayo Clinic's perspective on therapeutics, I will cover both of these along with other notions for how to get better when you catch COVID-19. We'll get there soon

Lagevrio and Paxlovid are similar to an extent. Both medications are authorized for high-risk people. My sisters are above seventy years of age and so that makes them the right candidates. The medicine should be started within 5 days of first feeling symptoms of COVID-19. There are several similarities between Paxlovid and molnupiravir. But the biggest difference lies in how effective they've been at treating COVID-19 in studies.

What is Paxlovid?

Paxlovid is the name used by doctors when prescribing this therapeutic manufactured by Pfizer. It is a combination of two antiviral pills: nirmatrelvir and ritonavir. Historically, it was the first oral medication to receive FDA emergency use authorization (EUA) for treating mild to moderate COVID-19. Most of us remember when Hydroxychloroquine had the EUA back in the Trump days.

Paxlovid is authorized for adults and children ages 12 and older who weigh at least 88 pounds (40 kg). The target audience for drugs like this often changes with more experience over time. Paxlovid is currently only recommended for people at high risk of developing severe COVID-19. High-risk people include older adults and those with certain medical conditions.

The manufacturer says here is how Paxlovid works to treat COVID-19?

Remember it is a combination medicine. The two medications in Paxlovid, nirmatrelvir and ritonavir, work together to help treat COVID-19. They both belong to the same class of medications known as protease inhibitors.

Nirmatrelvir stops the virus that causes COVID-19 from copying itself. The virus relies on an enzyme (protein) in our bodies called protease and it uses it to copy itself. Nirmatrelvir temporarily stops this enzyme from working so the virus can't use it to multiply. These are both key elements as to why this works.

Ritonavir helps to slow the breakdown of nirmatrelvir. This helps nirmatrelvir stay in the body at higher levels for a longer period of time. In other words, ritonavir helps make nirmatrelvir more effective against COVID-19 than it would be on its own. As you can tell, the experts in this case sure seem to know what they are doing.

What is Molnupiravir? It is also called Lagevrio which Is what my sister received.

Lagevrio/ Molnupiravir is also an oral antiviral pill that has been authorized to treat mild to moderate COVID-19. This medication, is manufactured by Merck. It received its EUA shortly after Paxlovid.

Lagevrio/ Molnupiravir is authorized in the EUA for adults ages 18 and older who are at high risk of developing severe COVID-19. However, the FDA has stated that Lagevrio/ Molnupiravir should only be used if no other recommended COVID-19 treatments are available. So, that does not explain why one sister received Paxlovid and the other Lagevrio/ Molnupiravir.

How does Lagevrio/ Molnupiravir work in fighting for COVID-19?

Lagevrio/ Molnupiravir is a nucleoside analog antiviral. It also stops the COVID-19 virus from copying itself, but it does this in a different way than Paxlovid. Lagecrio/ Molnupiravir looks like the genetic building blocks that the COVID-19 virus uses to copy itself.

So when you take the medication, the virus mistakenly inserts molnupiravir into its genetic material. When this happens, the virus can't copy itself. These researchers who figure this stuff out are very smart.

To summarize, it helps to remember that Paxlovid is an oral antiviral pill that can be taken at home to help keep high-risk patients from getting so sick that they need to be hospitalized. So, if you test positive for the coronavirus and you are eligible to take the pills, you can take them at home and lower your risk of going to the hospital.

Likewise it helps to know that Lagevrio / Molnupiravir is an investigational medicine used to treat mild-to-moderate COVID-19 in adults: with positive results of direct SARS-CoV-2 viral testing, and

• who are at high risk for progression to severe COVID-19 including hospitalization or death, and for whom other COVID-19 treatment options approved or authorized are not available

A further perspective on Lagevrio is given by EMA's human medicines committee (CHMP). It has issued advice on the use of Lagevrio (also known as molnupiravir or MK 4482) for the treatment of COVID-19. This medicine, which is currently not authorised in the EU, can be used to treat adults with COVID-19 who do not require supplemental oxygen and who are at increased risk of developing severe COVID-19. Lagevrio should be administered as soon as possible after diagnosis of COVID-19 and within 5 days of the start of symptoms. The medicine, which is available as capsules, should be taken twice a day for 5 days.

The Mayo Clinic Offers its Thoughts

As many of us have observed, the mud about therapeutics is thick and so the general public has been asking questions:

COVID-19 drugs: Are there any that work?

Among others, the Mayo Clinic from Rochester Minnesota has decided to weigh in and offer its thoughts on a plethora of solutions available for treatment

Questions come in often in the form of: "I've heard several drugs mentioned as possible treatments for COVID-19. What are they and how do they work?"

This is an answer to that question from Daniel C. DeSimone, M.D.

There is only one approved by the U.S. Food and Drug Administration (FDA) to treat coronavirus disease 2019 (COVID-19).

But many medications are being tested and evaluated.

Early on in COVID history, the FDA decided to approve an antiviral drug called Remdesivir (Veklury). It is targeted to treat COVID-19 in adults and children who are age 12 and older. It may be prescribed for people who are hospitalized with COVID-19 and need supplemental oxygen or have a higher risk of serious illness. It's given through a needle in the skin (intravenously). It is not available as an oral medication.

We just had a discussion about Paxlovid and Lagevrio/ Molnupiravi. Well, the Mayo Clinic again offers its perspective. If you already know this information from learning it in this chapter, that is great. Have patience there is new material offered by Mayo.

The FDA has authorized for emergency use a drug called Paxlovid. This drug combines two types of medications in one package. The first drug is nirmatrelvir. It blocks the activity of a specific enzyme needed for the virus that causes COVID-19 to replicate. The second drug is an antiviral drug called ritonavir. It helps slow the breakdown of nirmatrelvir. Paxlovid is authorized to treat mild to moderate COVID-19 in people age 12 and older who are at higher risk of serious illness.

These medications are taken by mouth as pills.

The FDA has also authorized for emergency use another drug called molnupiravir to treat mild to moderate COVID-19 in adults who are at higher risk of serious illness and not able to take other treatments. The medication is also taken by mouth as a pill.

The FDA has also authorized for emergency use the rheumatoid arthritis drug baricitinib (Olumiant) to treat COVID-19 in some cases. Baricitinib is a pill that seems to work against COVID-19 by reducing inflammation and having antiviral activity. Baricitinib may be used in people who are hospitalized with COVID-19 who are on mechanical ventilators or need supplemental oxygen.

Researchers are continually studying other potential treatments for COVID-19, including the following:

Antiviral drugs. Researchers are testing the antiviral drugs favipiravir and merimepodib. A number of studies have found that the combination of lopinavir and ritonavir is not effective.

Anti-inflammatory therapy. Researchers study many anti-inflammatory drugs to treat or prevent dysfunction of several organs and lung injury from infection-associated inflammation.

Dexamethasone. The corticosteroid dexamethasone is one type of anti-inflammatory drug that researchers are studying to treat or prevent organ dysfunction and lung injury from inflammation. Studies have found that this drug reduces the risk of death by about 30% for people on ventilators and by about 20% for people who need supplemental oxygen.

Dexamethasone has the recommendation of The U.S. National Institutes of Health for people hospitalized with COVID-19 who are on mechanical ventilators or need supplemental oxygen. If dexamethasone is not available, other corticosteroids, such as prednisone, methylprednisolone or hydrocortisone, may be used. Dexamethasone and other corticosteroids may be harmful if given for less severe COVID-19 infection.

In some cases, the drugs remdesivir, tocilizumab or baricitinib may be given with dexamethasone in hospitalized people who are on mechanical ventilators or need supplemental oxygen.

Immune-based therapy. Researchers study immune-based therapies, including convalescent plasma, mesenchymal stem cells and monoclonal antibodies. Many of us have heard about Monoclonal antibodies are proteins created in a lab that can help the immune system fight off viruses.

Monoclonal antibody medications include sotrovimab; bebtelovimab; a combination of bamlanivimab and etesevimab; and a combination of casirivimab and imdevimab. Some monoclonal antibodies, including bamlanivimab and etesevimab and casirivimab and imdevimab, aren't effective against COVID-19 caused by the omicron variant. However, sotrovimab and bebtelovimab can be used to treat COVID-19 caused by the omicron variant.

These drugs are used to treat mild to moderate COVID-19 in people who have a higher risk of developing serious illness due to COVID-19. Treatment involves a single infusion given by a needle in the arm (intravenously) in an outpatient setting. To be most effective, these medications need to be given soon after COVID-19 symptoms start and before hospitalization.

[**Notation:** Somehow, unfortunately, there are always political issues -- In 2020, the prime example was Hydroxychloroquine. In 2021, it was Ivermectin. And then in early in 2022, it was monoclonal antibodies, which multiple early studies suggest are not effective against the now-dominant omicron variant. Yet, others swear by it. Well in early 2022, The Food and Drug Administration announced that it would halt emergency-use authorizations for two monoclonal antibody therapies, one made by Regeneron Pharmaceuticals and one by Eli Lilly. At least with these monoclonal antibodies, unlike hydroxychloroquine and ivermectin, there was evidence they were once quite effective; that's just not the situation we find ourselves in at this point. Too bad we cannot get the politics out of medicine.]

Researchers also study the use of a type of immune-based therapy called **convalescent plasma**. The FDA has authorized for emergency use convalescent plasma therapy to treat COVID-19.

Convalescent plasma is blood donated by people who've recovered from COVID-19. Convalescent plasma with high antibodies may be used to treat some hospitalized people with COVID-19 who are either early in their illness or have weakened immune systems.

Drugs being studied that have uncertain effectiveness. Researchers study amlodipine and losartan. But it's not yet known how effective these drugs may be in treating or preventing COVID-19. Famotidine isn't thought to be beneficial in treating COVID-19.

Ivermectin. The drug ivermectin, used to treat or prevent parasites in animals and in humans, isn't a drug used to treat viruses. [though many swear by it]

The FDA hasn't approved use of this drug to treat or prevent COVID-19. Taking large doses of this drug can cause serious harm. Don't use medications intended for animals on yourself to treat or prevent COVID-19.

Hydroxychloroquine and chloroquine.

These malaria drugs had been authorized for emergency use by the FDA during the COVID-19 pandemic. However, the FDA withdrew that authorization when data analysis showed that the drugs are not effective for treating COVID-19. They can also cause serious heart problems. [There are a number of contrary opinions]

Drugs to prevent COVID-19. Researchers are studying drugs to prevent COVID-19 before and after exposure to the virus.

The FDA has authorized for emergency use the monoclonal antibody combination of tixagevimab and cilgavimab (Evusheld) to prevent COVID-19 in some people with weakened immune systems or a history of severe reactions to a COVID-19 vaccine.

It's not known if any of these will prove to be effective against COVID-19. It's critical to complete medical studies to determine whether any of these medications are effective against COVID-19.

Remember, do not try these medications without a prescription and your health care provider's approval, even if you've heard that they may have promise. These drugs can have serious side effects. They're reserved for people who are seriously ill and under a health care provider's care. The science and the art of medicine should be reserved for qualified licensed practitioners.

CHAPTER 12

The Hydroxychloroquine & Ivermectin Debate

The regular people in American and that means most of us, during the course of the pandemic seem to have lost faith and trust in the CDC and the FDA regarding therapeutics and vaccines and mandates and masks etc. for COVID. It is to the point where many simply have chosen not to accept what the CDC, for example, calls its evidence-based recommendations.

From patients who have been vaccinated dying after being injected to those vaccinated as many as four times, and still getting COVID, there is a lot of room for doubt when the CDC and / or the FDA make guiding pronouncements.

Yes, there are more and more reasons to doubt the government's supposed science experts —namely the CDC and the FDA. Their being wrong much of the time is the #1 reason that most give for doubting these once revere, thought to be infallible, experts.

I am not affiliated with the medical community other than in my role as a patient. However, I read profusely and I research theories and hypotheses and I come to conclusions. Do not take what my suppositions and conclusions are as gospel. Always check with your doctor before you make a call on what therapeutic or vaccinations to take or not take. Do not take the word of a pretty analytic book author because just like many others, he is not an expert in medicine.

People concerned about COVID, who once bought into the CDC's supposed evidence-based recommendations "lock, stock, and barrel" now look elsewhere for advice. Whether it is about vaccinations, face masks, or therapeutics like Hydroxychloroquine, and Ivermectin, the general population has been turning to other ways to prevent and/or treat COVID infections, rather than going back to what once was the horse's mouth.

Hydroxychloroquine was the first therapeutic to meet the jaundiced eye of the CDC, the FDA, and even the NIH. We can also include in the crowd of skeptics, the WOKE media, the liberal / progressive establishment and of course the Left and any Democrat that wants to keep carrying their card. Then, the same somewhat sinister but definitely prejudiced forces descended upon Ivermectin, a drug that had been used effectively for years to treat certain parasitic infections in the intestines, like pinworms and strongyloides. Yeah, now we're talking—pinworms…humph!

Like Hydroxychloroquine, there have been clinical studies to assess the effect of ivermectin on SARS-CoV-2 virus (COVID-19) infections. Also like hydroxychloroquine, none of what the "experts call well-done trials" have shown definitive proof that it is effective. However, the same experts will go so far as to admit that "poorly done studies," do show possible benefits.

Besides the studies, there are doctors and health providers who swear by both remedies. They swear that their patients survived COVID only because of the existence of these two drugs and they see major benefits from their personal experience with patients. Besides these, there are positive reports from the many patients who have taken Ivermectin for COVID and loudly proclaim its benefits.

The experts in the CDC and elsewhere discount these testimonials as biased and claim that it may be due to the placebo effect. Remember the reason the CDC has fallen from grace is they claimed that vaccinations and vaccine mandates and two to three masks would keep us all safe. So, it is natural that they would line up against something that doctors who prescribe to patients say works for their patients. Who are you going to believe? – Your doctor or the CDC?

So, who are you going to call? Who are you going to believe? Ghostbusters went away as an effective source of truth and remedy for all ills after its II remake. But just as there is a crowd of Hydroxychloroquine and Ivermectin haters, already in 1984 with the original Ghostbusters, we learned that just being funny is not enough nowadays for the modern liberal skeptics.

The liberal world came after Ghostbusters as if it was a religiously conservative movie. Sound familiar. Think of the reaction these two therapeutics played to after Donald Trump, who probably could have starred in either of the Ghostbusters' movies, claimed that Hydroxychloroquine was effective for COVID. *Donald Trump!* The mere mention of his name still makes liberals go aghast. So, they preach that anything Trump says, even if it is the truth, cannot be believed. So, now who are you going to call, Ghostbusters or the CDC?

There is a new word on Ghostbusters that it is a celebration. In other words, the left has labeled this very funny movie as a conservative propaganda bust in the same fashion that they say that Hydroxychloroquine and Ivermectin are bad for your health.

Can you remember in your lifetime any sane advice you received from the left? In other words, they accuse Ghostbusters of Reagan-era market conservatism, of entrepreneurship and privatization, of profit motives initiative, all of which prove more capable and effective ...ctor power. I guess that's bad.

...onservatives agree and say that Ghostbusters is arguably one of ...better examples not only of conservative filmmaking, but to further ...olster that opinion,— in 2009, flagship conservative journal National Review named it among the best conservative movies ever made — but of popular political filmmaking, period. What is funny and a factor which does make the movie work so well is that its political ideas are embedded in its story, characters, and world, growing organically out of the cultural context in which they are presented.

After all, the original version was set in New York in the early 1980s and the film does follow a group of failed academics as they take out dubious high-interest loans in order to start a small business, worrying as they do that, unlike the university, the private sector will "expect results." Ahem! Will all analysis of movie plots in the future result in a conservative or liberal stamp.

Anyway, my point is that bias in movies and bias in medicine may seem the same and perhaps the root cause for the bias is the same but denying yourself a conservative movie is a lot different than denying yourself what may be, after having four vaccinations and catching COVID anyway, the one therapeutic that may save your life – even if Whoopi Goldberg disapproves.

When you read, even today, supposed expert opinions about Hydroxychloroquine and Ivermectin, you can almost hear the bias coming loud and clears such as "But the weak evidence showing a benefit for ivermectin and the 31 ongoing ivermectin studies are encouraging some to take Ivermectin to prevent and/or treat their COVID infections. The politicians recommending Ivermectin are also contributing to this unfounded use. For them, scientific evidence appears to only be valid when it supports their positions."

CHAPTER 13

Is there a Scientific Consensus on Therapeutics?

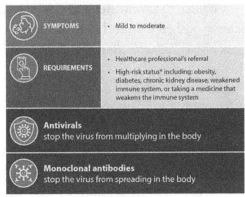

Hydroxychloroquine and Ivermectin

The answer is "no!" Ask Bret Weinstein

How many truths are there?

Bret Weinstein is what is termed an evolutionary biologist. He made headlines a while back when he was pressured out of his faculty position as a biology professor at Evergreen State College in Washington State because, guess what, he was accused of being a racist. No kidding. So how did that happen. Well, he opened his mouth and since it was in America, he felt he had a right to criticize an anti-White day of abstinence. Apparently not so.

If he was still in the left's good graces what he had to say to Tucker Carlson on Fox Nation may have been taken more seriously. Weinstein as a biologist had been analyzing the vaccines, and for his conclusions, he has summarily been censored for raising concerns about the shots and the medical establishment's opposition to alternative treatments such as Hydroxychloroquine, Ivermectin and others. It is simply not fair out there folks!

Weinstein decided to spill the beans on the anti-malarial drug Ivermectin so it would be approved as from his perspective, it has been proven effective against the coronavirus. Since it would minimize the usage of and potentially the ability to administer the U.S. coronavirus vaccines which are religiously pushed by the Food & Drug Administration's under an Emergency Use Authorization, the FDA et all are not rooting for it to succeed.

FYI, though Hydroxychloroquine earned its stripes for its effectiveness against malaria, Ivermectin is also an anti-malaria agent. We know that Malaria is transmitted through the bite of Plasmodium-infected adult female Anopheles mosquitoes. Ivermectin, properly characterized as an anti-parasitic drug, acts by killing mosquitoes that are exposed to the drug while feeding on the blood of people (known as blood feeds) who have ingested the drug. I say that serves the mosquito right! It suffers death in its last human blood feast.

In other words, Ivermectin may not be fully proven yet, but it is a good bet that the anecdotal studies and the results of patient use will eventually give it the green light or so it seems. Now it is not completely proven even yet. We know also that it is not good to cross the establishment when they have a stake in the outcome as government agencies are seemingly in beg with Big Pharma and oppose alternative treatments. So, Weinstein went from a bona fide liberal to Peck's Bad Boy overnight.

Here is some more on Weinstein. "If Ivermectin is what those of us who have looked at the evidence think it is, then the debate about the vaccines would be over by definition, because the vaccines that we have so far were granted emergency use authorization," Weinstein said. He also noted that the coronavirus vaccines are still not formally "approved" treatments by the FDA and instead have been and continue to be administered under the rarely-delineated category of EUA. Isn't that something.

Weinstein continues, according to the FDA's own definition, an EUA is "is a mechanism to facilitate the availability and use of medical countermeasures, including vaccines, during public health emergencies, such as the current COVID-19 pandemic."

"Under an EUA, the FDA may allow the use of unapproved medical products, or unapproved uses of approved medical products in an emergency to diagnose, treat, or prevent serious or life-threatening diseases or conditions when certain statutory criteria have been met, including that there are no adequate, approved, and available alternatives," the agency said.

Weinstein hangs his hat on the last clause of the agency's statement. He told Fox's Tucker Carlson, for example, that the clause is key to why it is important that Ivermectin and other established pharmaceuticals are thoroughly investigated as alternative treatments.

"That emergency use authorization has as a condition that there be no safe and effective treatments available," he said, noting that Ivermectin is old enough and established enough that it is "out of [its] patent" – meaning it can be produced generically – and has been proven safe and effective for other medical conditions. If you are scoring at home folks Weinstein struck a distinctive blow against the vaccines being the only EUA methods available.

We know from history that Ivermectin is not as time tested as Hydroxychloroquine, which has been around since the 1940's, but it too has been around for a lot of years—almost 50 years. It was discovered circa 1975 in Japan. It is most notably used as a treatment for malaria in the infested regions like Africa, and has also been used in veterinary medicine as a very common treatment for heartworm in domesticated dogs and cats. Ivermectin lotion has also been prescribed to treat head lice in children. It is not bad medicine folks but like all medicines, make sure your doctor approves.

Another reason on the plus side is that Ivermectin is a cost-effective medication for its current uses, with a 3-day prescription-withstanding supply costing less than $50 on Amazon. There you go! After you get your doctor's prescription, of course.

Weinstein did not stop there. Remember folks as an evolutionary Biologist, he is an expert in the field.

So, according to Weinstein, "If Ivermectin is safe and effective … then there shouldn't be vaccines that we're administering. They should be in testing and we should be finding out whether they are or are not safe," alluding to several serious cases of vaccine side effects.

Weinstein suggested that if the anti-malarial drugs are proven effective, it would moot the Emergency Use Authorization for the vaccine. In January,2022, the New York Post reported about a study of 573 patients administered Ivermectin for COVID. It revealed that only 8 individuals who received Ivermectin died versus 44 out of 510 who passed away after being administered a placebo.

It is never enough for the FDA so ask your doctor. Take the results of the study with you to his office. Why/ The FDA does not concur. In March they warned against Ivermectin's use as a treatment for COVID. Remember the drug has been used since 1975 to fight malaria.

But they claimed that "taking large doses of this drug is dangerous and can cause serious harm." The agency also warned that humans can be harmed if they ingest the derivative formulation of Ivermectin meant otherwise for dogs and horses. Well, why would anybody do that?

Fauci is not on Weinstein's side. The National Institutes of Health, (NIH) under which Dr. Anthony Fauci's NIAID falls, has offered its own take. They say "Ivermectin has been shown to inhibit the replication of SARS-CoV-2 [COVID-19 virus] in cell cultures," but that pharmacokinetic studies suggest "doses up to one-hundredfold higher" than approved anti-parasitic dosages in humans are needed to attain adequate treatment of coronavirus complications. Weinstein disagrees.

On "Tucker Carlson Today," Weinstein went on to lament that the U.S. and its federal medical bureaucracy appears to have no long-term plan to fight coronavirus, other than the potential for an unclear number of regular "booster shots" of the current COVID vaccine. The Biologist added that in the wake of strong adverse reactions, such as a Northern Virginia woman who suffered a massive brain-bleed, it is questionable why the establishment continues to expose Americans to vaccine risks, but folks, remember there is a lot of money -- $billions at stake.

There are the studies that have shown people who have been infected with COVID-19 have been "effectively vaccinated by the disease itself" and that that post-infection immunity is stronger and longer-lasting than vaccine-based resistance. If all human beings were honest, science would be science and not have all of the biases of humans looking for a big payoff. The message in all cases is to be careful what you take.

If you are looking for a safe bet, going against the establishment is not necessarily the right option, whether you think they tell the truth or not. The fact is that the US Food and Drug Administration (FDA) has not approved the use of either Hydroxychloroquine (HCQ) or Ivermectin for treating or preventing COVID-19 in humans.

Both drugs are FDA approved for other diseases and can be taken safely as directed by a doctor. Neither drug is officially classified as an anti-viral medication so technically if you go against the government, in essence, you are on your own. That is why it is so important for the public to use the advice of their own doctor.

Please know that I am not advocating that you go against your doctor's advice. Quite the contrary. This is information that to the best of my knowledge is accurate but I am again, not an expert. There does seem to be a lot of contrary opinions about Hydroxychloroquine and Ivermectin. Too bad science cannot form a consensus.

Here are some of the government's bad reports:

There are documented and studied dangers of using ivermectin

- Do not swallow ivermectin lotion or cream that is meant for use on the skin.
- Taking large doses or doses intended for animals is dangerous and can result in overdose, causing serious harm including nausea, vomiting, diarrhea, low blood pressure, dizziness, balance problems, seizures, coma, and even death.
- Ivermectin can cause birth defects if taken early in pregnancy.
- Dosages intended for animals may contain ingredients that are not meant for people to consume, and how these ingredients can affect humans has not been studied.

There are also documented and studied dangers of using hydroxychloroquine (HCQ)

- High quality research data show the use of HCQ for treating COVID-19 can be dangerous and has no medical benefit. In fact, the FDA has revoked emergency use authorization for HCQ in COVID-19 patients based on these dangers and because it does not help people recover faster.
- HCQ should not be taken for COVID-19 infection because it can cause serious heart rhythm abnormalities, severe liver inflammation, and kidney failure.

Some might say that if you get anything else out of this book, consider this: Taking HCQ on your own outside the hospital is dangerous. Please consult a qualified physician.

OTHER BOOKS BY BRIAN W. KELLY

Larry Elder Governor of California. Perfect candidate for California

WineDiets.Com Renews: The Wine Diet Includes three wine diets & an alcohol-free diet

Katie Kelly & Her Miracle Voice Singer, Songwriter, Musician and Producer

Beating Big Tech Monopolies! Just like when the Trustbusters beat the robber-barons in 1900s

The Great Story of Florida Gators Football Beginning of football to the Coach Dan Mullen's era

The Great Story of LSU Football The beginning of football to the Ed Orgeron era

The Great Story of Clemson Football Starts at the first football game to the Dabo Swinney era

The Great Story of Alabama Football From the first college football game to Alabama's last TD u

The Great Story of Notre Dame Football The beginning of football to coach Brian Kelly's last game

The Great Story of Penn State Football From the beginning of football to the last James Franklin game

Great Moments in College Football From the beginning of football to the 2020 post season.

Great Players in Tampa Bay Buccaneers Football From the beginning of football through the Bruce Ariens era

Super Bowl & NFL Championship Seasons: The Tampa Bay Buccaneers First championship to Super B

Great Coaches in Tampa Bay Buccaneers Football Begins continues through the Bruce Ariens era.

Great Moments in Tampa Bay Buccaneers Football Begins beginning of Football to Bruce Ariens era.

Donald Trump Governor of California After the Newsom recall, Trump is the perfect candidate

Ron DeSantis: The Best United States Governor To Governors what Trump is to Presidents—The Best!

Mike v Trump: Mike Grant takes on Donald Trump; Brian Kelly takes on Mike Grant;

SCOTUS Eliminatus No country needs a Supreme Court that refuses to hear critical cases!

The Corruption in the WB Area School District A Story about toxic corruption and other stinky things

Stolen Election ??? Democrats say: "fair and just;" Republicans surrender to Democrats

The Ten Commandments of Calipered Kinematically Aligned Total Knee Arthroplasty Color

The Ten Commandments of Calipered Kinematically Aligned Total Knee Arthroplasty B/W

About Alexa! Tell me how!

Chronicle of Inept Governance & Corrective Actions board from hell big question: better way?

Hey Alexa Create me my own personal musical paradise Unnpublished with new book

FTC Case: LetsGoPublish.com v Amazon Fourth Edition big bully censored nine books

FTC Case: LetsGoPublish.com v Amazon Third Edition big bully censored nine books

FTC Case: LetsGoPublish.com v Amazon Second Edition big bully censored nine books

The President Donald J. Trump Book Catalog Color Version by Brian Kelly & Lets Go Publish!

The President Donald J. Trump Book Catalog B/W Version by Brian Kelly & Lets Go Publish!

FTC Case: LetsGoPublish.com v Amazon Original case bully censored nine books

What America Wins if Biden Wins Everything!!!!!! The answer is really nothing.

What America Loses if Trump Loses None of the 1000s of Trump wins for starters

What America Wins When Trump Wins Trump already gave the country more benefits and blessings

We Love Trump! Don't you? The President given to the people by God as the answer to our prayers

Amazon: The Biggest Bully in Town bully blocked eight books in 2020 by most published author

Trump Assured 2020 Victory President needs these two prongs for his platform for landslide

2020 Republican Convention—Speeches Blocked by Amazon Includes memento free Link

2020 RNC Convention Full Speech Transcripts Blocked by Amazon Memento of the 87 best

COVID-19 Mask, Yes? Or No? It's Everybody's Recommended Solution!!!

LSU Tigers Championship Seasons Starts at beginning of LSU Football to the National Championship

Great Coaches in LSU Football Book starts with the first LSU coach; goes to Orgeron Championship

Great Players in LSU Football Begins with 1893 QB Ruffin G Pleasant to 2019 QB Burrow

America for Millennialsl A growing # of disintegrationists want to tear US down

Great Moments in LSU Football Book starts at start of Football to the Ed Orgeron Championship.

The Constitution's Role in a Return to Normalcy Can the Constitution Survive?

The Constitution vs. The Virus Simultaneous attack coronavirus and US governors

One, Two, Three, Pooph!!! Reopen Country Now! Return to normalcy is just around the corner.

Reopen America Now Return to Normalcy

Enough is Enough!Re Re: Covid, We are not children. We're adults.We'll make the right decisions.

How to Write Your 1st Book & Publish it Using Amazon KDP You can do it

REMDESIVIR A Ray of Hope

When Will America Reopen for Business? This author's opinion includes voices of experts

HydroxyChloroquine: The Game Changer

Super Bowl & NFL Championship Seasons The KC Chiefs From the 1st to Super Bowl LIV

Great Coaches in Kansas City Chiefs Football First Coach era to Andy Reid Era

Great Players in Kansas City Chiefs Football From the AFL to Andy Reid Era

Reopen America Now! How to Shut-Down Corona Virus & Return to Normalcy!

Why is Everybody Moving to the Villages? You can afford a home in the Villages

CORONAVIRUS The Cause & the Cure. Many solutions—but which ones will work?

Great Moments in Kansas City Chiefs Football. From the beginning to the Andy Reid Era

How the Philadelphia Eagles Lost Its Karma. This is the one place that tells the story

Cancel All Student Debt Now! Good for America, Good for the Economy.

Social Security Screw Job!!! Scandal: Seniors Intentionally Screwed by US Government

Trump Hate They hate Trump Supporters; Trump; & God—in that order

Christmas Wings for Brian A heartwarming story of a boy whose shoulders kept growing

Merry Christmas to Wilkes-Barre 50 Ways" for Mayor George Brown to Create a Better City.

Air Force Football Championship Seasons From AF Championship to Coach Calhoun's latest team

Syracuse Football Championship Seasons beginning of SU championships; goes to Dino Babers Era

Navy Football Championship Seasons 1st Navy Championships to the Ken Niumatalolo Era

Army Football Championship Seasons Beginning of Football championships to Jeff Monken Era

Florida Gators Championship Seasons Beginning of Football through championships to Dan Mullen era

Alabama's Championship Seasons Beginning of Football past the 2017/2018 National Championship

Clemson Tigers Championship Seasons Beginning of Football to the Clemson National Championships

Penn State's Championship Seasons PSU's first championship to the James Franklin era

Notre Dame's Championship Seasons Before Knute Rockne and past Lou Holtz's 1988 undisputed title

Super Bowls & Championship Seasons: The New York Giants Many championships of the Giants.

Super Bowls & Championship Seasons: New England Patriots Many championships of the Patriots.

Super Bowls & Championship Seasons: The Pittsburgh Steelers Many championship of the Steelers

Super Bowls & Championship Seasons: The Philadelphia Eagles Many championships of the Eagles.

The Big Toxic School Wilkes-Barre Area's Tale of Corruption, Deception, Taxation & Tyranny

Great Players in New York Giants Football Begins with great players of 1925 to the Saquon Barqley era.

Great Coaches in New York Giants Football Begins with Bob Folwell 1925 and to Pat Shurmur in 2019.

Great Moments in New York Giants Football Beginning of Football to the Pat Shurmur era.

Hasta La Vista California Give California its independence.

IT's ALL OVER! Mueller: NO COLLUSION!"—Top Dems going to jail for the hoax!

Democrat Secret for Power & Winning Elections Open borders adds millions of new Democrat Voters

Hope for Wilkes-Barre—John Q. Doe—Next Mayor of Wilkes-Barre

The John Doe Plan & WB Plan will help create a better city!

Great Moments in New England Patriots Football Second Edition

This book begins at the beginning of Football and goes to the Bill Belichick era.

The Cowardly Congress Corrupt US Congress is against America and Americans.

Great Players in Air Force Football From the beginning to the current season

Great Coaches in Air Force Football Grom the beginning to Coach Troy Calhoun

Help for Mayor George and Next Mayor of Wilkes-Barre How to vote for the next Mayor Council

Ghost of Wilkes-Barre Future: Spirit's advice for residents how to pick the next Mayor and Council

Great Players in Air Force Football: Air Force's best players of all time

Great Coaches in Air Force Football: From Coach 1 to Coach Troy Calhoun

Great Moments in Air Force Football: From day 1 to today

Great Players in Navy Football: Navy's best including Bellino & Staubach

Great Coaches in Navy Football: From Coach 1 to Coach #39 Ken Niumatalolo

Great Moments in Navy Football: From day 1 to coach Ken Niumatalolo 1

No Tree! No Toys! No Toot! Heartwarming story. Christmas gone while 19 month old napped

How to End DACA, Sanctuary Cities, & Resident Illegal Aliens. best solution remove shadowsAmerica.

Government Must Stop Ripping Off Seniors' Social Security!: Hey buddy, seniors can't spare a dime?

Special Report: Solving America's Student Debt Crisis!: The only real solution to the $1.52 Trillion debt

The Winning Political Platform for America Unique winning approach to solve big problems in America.

Lou Barletta v Bob Casey for US Senate Barletta's unique approach to solve big problems in America.

John Chrin v Matt Cartwright for Congress Chrin has a unique approach to solve big problems in America.

The Cure for Hate !!! Can the cure be any worse than this disease that is crippling America?

Andrew Cuomo's Time to Go? He Was Never that Great!": Cuomo says America never that great

White People Are Bad! Bad! Bad! Whoever thought a popular slogan in 2018 It's OK to be White!

The Fake News Media Is Also Corrupt !!!: Fake press / media today is not worthy to be 4th Estate.

God Gave US Donald Trump? Trump was sent from God as the people's answer

Millennials Say America Was Never That Great": Too many pleased days of political chumps not over!

It's Time for The John Q. Doe Party… Don't you think? By Elephants.

Great Players in Florida Gators Football… Tim Tebow and a ton of other great players

Great Coaches in Florida Gators Football… The best coaches in Gator history.

The Constitution by Hamilton, Jefferson, Madison, et al. The Real Constitution

The Constitution Companion. Will help you learn and understand the Constitution

Great Coaches in Clemson Football The best Clemson Coaches right to Dabo Swinney

Great Players in Clemson Football The best Clemson players in history

Winning Back America. America's been stolen and can be won back completely

The Founding of America... Great book to pick up a lot of great facts

Defeating America's Career Politicians. The scoundrels need to go.

Midnight Mass by Jack Lammers... You remember what it was like Great story

The Bike by Jack Lammers... Great heartwarming Story by Jack

Wipe Out All Student Loan Debt--Now! Watch the economy go boom!

No Free Lunch Pay Back Welfare! Why not pay it back?

Deport All Millennials Now!!! Why they deserve to be deported and/or saved

DELETE the EPA, Please! The worst decisions to hurt America

Taxation Without Representation 4th Edition Should we throw the TEA overboard again?

Four Great Political Essays by Thomas Dawson

Top Ten Political Books for 2018... Cliffnotes Version of 10 Political Books

Top Six Patriotic Books for 2018... Cliffnotes version of 6 Patriotic Boosk

Why Trump Got Elected!. It's great to hear about a great milestone in America!

The Day the Free Press Died. Corrupt Press Lives on!

Solved (Immigration) The best solutions for 2018

Solved II (Obamacare, Social Security, Student Debt) Check it out; They're solved.

Great Moments in Pittsburgh Steelers Football... Six Super Bowls and more.

Great Players in Pittsburgh Steelers Football,,,Chuck Noll, Bill Cowher, Mike Tomin, etc.

Great Coaches in New England Patriots Football,,, Bill Belichick the one and only plus others

Great Players in New England Patriots Football... Tom Brady, Drew Bledsoe et al.

Great Coaches in Philadelphia Eagles Football..Andy Reid, Doug Pederson & Lots more

Great Players in Philadelphia Eagles Football Great players such as Sonny Jurgenson

Great Coaches in Syracuse Football All the greats including Ben Schwartzwalder

Great Players in Syracuse Football. Highlights best players such as Jim Brown & Donovan McNabb

Millennials are People Too !!! Give US millennials help to live American Dream

Brian Kelly for the United States Senate from PA: Fresh Face for US Senate

The Candidate's Bible. Don't pray for your campaign without this bible

Rush Limbaugh's Platform for Americans… Rush will love it

Sean Hannity's Platform for Americans… Sean will love it

Donald Trump's New Platform for Americans. Make Trump unbeatable in 2020

Tariffs Are Good for America! One of the best tools a president can have

Great Coaches in Pittsburgh Steelers Football Sixteen of the best coaches ever to coach in pro football.

Great Moments in New England Patriots Football Great football moments from Boston to New England

Great Moments in Philadelphia Eagles Football. The best from the Eagles from the beginning of football.

Great Moments in Syracuse Football The great moments, coaches & players in Syracuse Football

Boost Social Security Now! Hey Buddy Can You Spare a Dime?

The Birth of American Football. From the first college game in 1869 to the last Super Bowl

Obamacare: A One-Line Repeal Congress must get this done.

A Wilkes-Barre Christmas Story A wonderful town makes Christmas all the better

A Boy, A Bike, A Train, and a Christmas Miracle A Christmas story that will melt your heart

Pay-to-Go America-First Immigration Fix

Legalizing Illegal Aliens Via Resident Visas Americans-first plan saves $Trillions. Learn how!

60 Million Illegal Aliens in America!!! A simple, America-first solution.

The Bill of Rights By Founder James Madison Refresh your knowledge of the specific rights for all

Great Players in Army Football Great Army Football played by great players..

Great Coaches in Army Football Army's coaches are all great.

Great Moments in Army Football Army Football at its best.

Great Moments in Florida Gators Football Gators Football from the start. This is the book.

Great Moments in Clemson Football CU Football at its best. This is the book.

Great Moments in Florida Gators Football Gators Football from the start. This is the book.

The Constitution Companion. A Guide to Reading and Comprehending the Constitution

The Constitution by Hamilton, Jefferson, & Madison – Big type and in English

PATERNO: The Dark Days After Win # 409. Sky began to fall within days of win # 409.

JoePa 409 Victories: Say No More! Winningest Division I-A football coach ever

American College Football: The Beginning From before day one football was played.

Great Coaches in Alabama Football Challenging the coaches of every other program!

Great Coaches in Penn State Football the Best Coaches in PSU's football program

Great Players in Penn State Football The best players in PSU's football program

Great Players in Notre Dame Football The best players in ND's football program

Great Coaches in Notre Dame Football The best coaches in any football program

Great Players in Alabama Football from Quarterbacks to offensive Linemen Greats!

Great Moments in Alabama Football AU Football from the start. This is the book.

Great Moments in Penn State Football PSU Football, start--games, coaches, players,

Great Moments in Notre Dame Football ND Football, start, games, coaches, players

Cross Country with the Parents A great trip from East Coast to West with the kids

Seniors, Social Security & the Minimum Wage. Things seniors need to know.

How to Write Your First Book and Publish It with CreateSpace. You too can be an author.

The US Immigration Fix--It's all in here. Finally, an answer.

I had a Dream IBM Could be #1 Again The title is self-explanatory

WineDiets.Com Presents The Wine Diet Learn how to lose weight while having fun.

Wilkes-Barre, PA; Return to Glory Wilkes-Barre City's return to glory

Geoffrey Parsons' Epoch... The Land of Fair Play Better than the original.

The Bill of Rights 4 Dummmies! This is the best book to learn about your rights.

Sol Bloom's Epoch …Story of the Constitution The best book to learn the Constitution

America 4 Dummmies! All Americans should read to learn about this great country.

The Electoral College 4 Dummmies! How does it really work?

The All-Everything Machine Story about IBM's finest computer server.

ThankYou IBM! This book explains how IBM was beaten in the computer marketplace by neophytes

Amazon.com/author/brianwkelly

Brian W. Kelly has written 309 books including this book.

Thanks again for buying this one.

www.ingramcontent.com/pod-product-compliance
Lightning Source LLC
Chambersburg PA
CBHW021614310125
21206CB00020B/53